BODY CONDITIONING FOR COLLEGE MEN

ALFRED E. SCHOLZ

and

ROBERT E. JOHNSON

Instructors in the Department of Physical
Education, Yale University

ILLUSTRATED BY VERNON HÜPPI

W. B. SAUNDERS COMPANY

PHILADELPHIA • LONDON • TORONTO

W. B. Saunders Company: West Washington Square
Philadelphia, Pa. 19105

12 Dyott Street
London W.C.1

1835 Yonge Street
Toronto 7, Ontario

GV
481
.S28
1969

Saunders Physical Activities Series

Body Conditioning for College Men

© 1969 by W. B. Saunders Company. Copyright under the International Copyright Union. All rights reserved. This book is protected by copyright. No part of it may be reproduced or duplicated in any manner without written permission from the publisher. Made in the United States of America. Press of W. B. Saunders Company. Library of Congress catalog card number 69-17804.

EDITORS' FOREWORD

Every period of history, as well as every society, has its own profile. Our own world of the last third of the twentieth century is no different. Whenever we step back to look at ourselves, we can see excellences and failings, strengths and weaknesses, that are peculiarly ours.

One of our strengths as a nation is that we are a sports-loving people. Today more persons—and not just young people—are playing, watching, listening to, and reading about sports and games. Those who enjoy themselves most are the men and women who actually *play* the game: the "doers."

You are reading this book now for either of two very good reasons. First, you want to learn—whether in a class or on your own—how to play a sport well, and you need clear, easy-to-follow instructions to develop the special skills involved. If you want to be a successful player, this book will be of much help to you.

Second, you may already have developed skill in this activity, but want to improve your performance through assessing your weaknesses and correcting your errors. You want to develop further the skills you have now and to learn and perfect additional ones. You realize that you will enjoy the activity even more if you know more about it.

In either case, this book can contribute greatly to your success. It offers "lessons" from a real professional: from an outstandingly successful coach, teacher, or performer. All the authors in the *Saunders Physical Activities Series* are experts and widely recognized in their specialized fields. Some have been members or coaches of teams of national prominence and Olympic fame.

This book, like the others in our Series, has been written to make it easy for you to help yourself to learn. The authors and the editors want you to become more self-motivated and to gain a greater understanding of, appreciation for, and proficiency in the exciting world of *movement*. All the activities described in this Series—sports, games, dance, body conditioning, and weight and figure control activities—require skillful, efficient movement. That's what physical activity is all about. Each book contains descriptions and helpful tips about the nature, value, and purpose of an activity, about the purchase and care of equipment, and about the fundamentals of each movement skill involved. These books also tell you about common errors and how to avoid making them, about ways in which you can improve your performance, and about game rules and strategy, scoring, and special techniques. Above all, they should tell you how to get the most pleasure and benefit from the time you spend.

Our purpose is to make you a successful *participant* in this age of sports activities. If you are successful, you will participate often—and this will give you countless hours of creative and recreative fun. At the same time, you will become more physically fit.

"Physical fitness" is more than just a passing fad or a slogan. It is a condition of your body which determines how effectively you can perform your daily work and play and how well you can meet unexpected demands on your strength, your physical skills, and your endurance. How fit you are depends largely on your participation in vigorous physical activity. Of course no one sports activity can provide the kind of total workout of the body required to achieve optimal fitness; but participation with vigor in any activity makes a significant contribution to this total. Consequently, the activity you will learn through reading this book can be extremely helpful to you in developing and maintaining physical fitness now and throughout the years to come.

These physiological benefits of physical activity are important beyond question. Still, the pure pleasure of participation in physical activity will probably provide your strongest motivation. The activities taught in this Series are *fun*, and they provide a most satisfying kind of recreation for your leisure hours. Also they offer you great personal satisfaction in achieving success in skillful performance —in the realization that you are able to control your body and its movement and to develop its power and beauty. Further, there can be a real sense of fulfillment in besting a skilled opponent or in exceeding a goal you have set for yourself. Even when you fall short of such triumphs, you can still find satisfaction in the effort you have made to meet a challenge. By participating in sports you can gain greater respect for yourself, for others, and for "the rules of the game." Your skills in leadership and fellowship will be sharpened and improved. Last, but hardly least, you will make new friends among others who enjoy sports activities, both as participants and as spectators.

We know you're going to enjoy this book. We hope that it—and the others in our Series—will make you a more skillful and more enthusiastic performer in all the activities you undertake.

Good luck!

MARYHELEN VANNIER

HOLLIS FAIT

PREFACE

In these days of uncertainty and great tension, it might be well for us to be less concerned with adding years to our life, since that is not always within our power, but to be, instead, more concerned with the many bountiful physical benefits to be derived from exercise, which can add life to our years. It is this concept of the value of exercise that has guided the preparation and presentation of the materials in this text.

The discussion of the benefits and values of exercise, supported by numerous statements from prominent medical doctors, health specialists, nutritionists and physical fitness leaders, is directed toward motivating the reader to begin a program of body conditioning. To help him start his program, exercise routines for daily workouts are presented in detail. These can be performed simply, with a minimum of equipment, space and preliminary preparation. Fundamental exercise plans and charts are presented in clear, concise fashion for easy, effective use by the novice.

It is recognized that those who use this book will differ greatly in their basic conditioning needs and in the goals they desire to achieve. They will range from those with very poor levels of physical fitness to superbly conditioned athletes who are interested primarily in improving their ability in performing a certain sport. The organization of the units presenting various types of conditioning exercises will enable each individual to choose a plan or exercise routine that best fits his needs and goals. For determining how much progress he is making in improving his physical fitness, there are included quick and simple self-evaluation tests.

The temptation to use a new vocabulary when writing about a familiar subject is very appealing, especially when the subject is timely and is constantly before the public, as physical fitness is today. The terms energy, calories of work, figure control, graded programs, aerobics and dynamic tension all have more appeal than the words calisthenics, conditioning and exercise. The simple truth is, however, that an elbow, knee or hip joint flexes in only one direction and extends in the opposite direction. Such movements require work; the harder we work, the more energy we expend and the more demands we place upon the body. Once the body begins to respond to the demands, the gateway to high physical efficiency has been entered. Newer and fancier terms do not change either the results or the process by which they are achieved. Therefore, the authors have resisted temptation and have employed the old familiar terms.

PRESIDENTIAL MESSAGES*

Experience has taught me that regular exercise, proper diet and adequate rest and relaxation are essential to good health. I swim twice daily; I enjoy walking in the outdoors.

Physical activity provides relief from tension, and it also builds the strength and endurance all of us need.

America's young men and women are taller, heavier and healthier than ever before. They can be the most energetic and productive citizens in the world. This is a challenge which I know each of you will want to help meet.

Fourteen percent of our children still do not participate in any physical activity programs at all, and another 27 percent take part only one or two days a week. Our goals in these years ahead certainly should be 100 percent participation.

Every adult should find time in his daily schedule for some form of physical activity. Medical evidence tells us that our heart, lungs, muscles and even our minds need the effects of regular and vigorous exercise.

Overweight and flagging stamina, the badges of the unfit, now are recognized as invitations to old age and illness.

Despite the comfort of modern existence, life still demands the best that we can give. Leisure must not mean physical inactivity and idleness. Instead, we must recognize it as an opportunity to strengthen and refresh ourselves for our roles as creative and productive citizens.

---

*Former President Lyndon B. Johnson, quoted from publications of the President's Council on Physical Fitness.

There is no question but what the health and physical fitness of their students is a proper concern for institutions of higher education. It is only in the hands of those who have the energy, skill and courage to use it well that knowledge can expand men and societies.

As a former teacher, I understand the problems our colleges and universities face—limited human and material resources to do an unlimited and urgent task. An important part of this task is assuring that our most able and best trained young people also have that degree of physical fitness that will enable them to lead full and productive lives.

WHY EXERCISE

Modern civilization is tending to shape man into a nervous, tense individual who has very few demands made upon him for vigorous physical exertion. The need for exercise has been emphasized by Presidents Eisenhower, Kennedy, and Johnson, through the channels of the President's Council on Physical Fitness. The presidential messages of Mr. Johnson and the many quotations of authorities on the subject, whose statements are listed below, lend support to the idea that a basic need of man is to perform physical work. Exercise, especially that which is prescribed by experienced technicians in the field, can satisfy the need and serve as a substitute for that physical work.

Exercise helps to relieve tension. It will increase your strength, flexibility, agility and endurance. By exercising you will feel better, look better, and work more efficiently. By exercising regularly, it is possible with proper diet to gain weight, lose weight, or maintain a consistent weight. Some of the latest articles written on jogging and running suggest that the incidence of heart failure can be reduced by this form of exercise, thereby increasing the life span of many potential coronary victims.

C. E. Turner, Dr. P.H., former President of the International Union for Health Education of the Public, says, "Young persons need a well-planned program of physical exercise if they are to secure an all-around physical development . . . The beneficial effects of muscular exercise include: (1) an aid to circulation, (2) an increase in red corpuscles and hemoglobin, (3) an aid in the removal of waste from tissues, (4) clearing the skin, (5) strengthening the muscular system, (6) aiding digestion, (7) improving the mental tone, (8) relieving internal congestion, (9) strengthening and enlarging the lungs, and (10) strengthening the heart.

Ernst Jokl, M.D., urges regular exercise as "preventive medicine": "Those who maintain activity have better performance records, less degenerative diseases and probably a longer life expectancy than the general population" . . . "There is little doubt but that the proper physical activity as a part of a way of life can significantly delay the aging process."

C. Ward Crampton, M.D. "We need the effects of muscular exercise on the internal organs, for it is only through big muscular work that we can strengthen the heart, lungs, liver, intestines and endocrine organs. Pills will not do it, neither will massage, nor yet faith, for faith without work is dead."

Howard B. Sprague, M.D., a noted Boston heart specialist, feels that, along with proper diet, "The best insurance against coronary disease is exercise—lots of it. By walking at least two miles a day you are building up an accessory circulation for that inevitable coronary."

Jean Mayer, Ph.D., D.S.C. "Exercise should be graded according to age, individual reaction to activity and the state of the person's fitness. After the age of forty, more frequent medical evaluation of the individual capacity for exercise is imperative."

Peter Karpovitch, M.D. "A low degree of fitness seems inadvisable as it leaves no margin of safety for the experiences of adversity which frequently descend upon mankind."

Warren G. Guild, M.D. "Anyone past the age of thirty who wants to keep fit should have two objectives. He must choose a sport in which stamina, not speed, is the object—avoiding short spurts of work, and he must pursue it with regularity, not merely on weekends. A half-hour a day of exercise for six days a week will get you in awfully good shape and it will reduce your susceptibility in the degenerative diseases."

Lawrence Morehouse, Ph.D., and Augustus Miller, M.D. "One of the most fundamental of physiologic laws is that functional efficiency of an organ or system improves with use and regresses with disuse."

Jesse Feiring William, M.D. "Habituation to physical activities is one of the goals that should be set not only for every college man and woman but for all persons in the formative periods of life."

J. Roswell Gallagher, M.D. "Remember, to be sufficiently fit to do the unusual allows one to perform mild exertion with little cost."

Walter McClellan, Ph.D. "A regular plan of physical exercise properly followed through young adulthood and middle age, I believe, will provide the older person with a better physical machine."

Morris Fishbein, M.D. "Following a reasonable amount of exercise in the open air, the body feels refreshed and not exhausted. With such refreshment comes the relaxation that is exceedingly important for rest and good mental hygiene."

CONTENTS

Unit I

An Introduction to Exercise	1
Physical Fitness	3
Principles of Weight Reduction	6
Height – Weight – Body Build Standards (For Both Sexes)	7

Unit II

How to Begin	10
Circuit Training	11
The First Dozen	15
An Evaluation	28
The Second Dozen	28

Unit III

New Trends in Exercise	43
The Big Ten: Isometrics	44
A Busy Man's Special	54
Weight Training	57
Flexibility Exercise	68
Pulley Weight Exercise	72

Unit IV

Evaluation	75
The Yale Tests	78
AAHPER Tests	85
The Sigma Delta Psi Test	87

Unit V

TRAINING FOR ENDURANCE	90
RUNNING AND JOGGING	90
SWIMMING	95
STAIR CLIMBING	96
BENCH STEPPING	96
BICYCLING	96
ROWING	97

Unit VI

CONDITIONING FOR SPORTS	98
SPECIFIC SPORTS EXERCISES	98
CONDITIONING THROUGH RECREATION	109

GLOSSARY	112
BIBLIOGRAPHY	114

UNIT I

AN INTRODUCTION TO EXERCISE
PHYSICAL FITNESS
PRINCIPLES OF WEIGHT REDUCTION
HEIGHT AND WEIGHT CHART

AN INTRODUCTION TO EXERCISE

Great fortunes are expended annually for the upkeep of homes, factories, office buildings, churches, automobiles and boats. Great pride is taken in their attractive appearance, and the time given to maintaining them in top condition is considered well spent. It is ironical that people who lavish so much money, time and effort on the upkeep and care of material possessions concern themselves so little with the condition of their bodies. Unless injury or illness occurs, they usually give little thought to maintaining an efficient, healthy body. The ancient Greeks regarded the body as the temple of the mind and gave it the respectful care due such a "building." If we moderns were to hold the body in the same high regard and devote to its care and upkeep a fair allotment of the time and effort now given our material possessions, we would undoubtedly be more fit, physically and mentally, to cope with the stresses and strains of our environment and to enjoy life more fully.

One of the most important means of maintaining the efficiency and fitness of the body is regular systematic exercise; that is, a definite plan of exercise that will ensure total body workout. In this way all major muscle groups will receive appropriate exercise to develop strength, speed, power and endurance, which are some of the components of physical fitness.

The heart and lungs are required to work harder during exercise and, as a result, cardiorespiratory endurance (another component of physical fitness) is increased. The selected exercises must be engaged in on a regular basis, however, for in order to improve the level of physical fitness the strenuousness of the workout must be continually increased over a period of time. Once the desired level of physical fitness is reached the exertion levels off; but any decrease in the work load will cause a decrease in the fitness level of the body.

When muscles are not used, a decrease in strength, efficiency and size results. This is true of the muscles of the organs of the body, such as the heart, as well as of the skeletal muscles. The condition resulting from the lack of use is called atrophy. Severe atrophy results in muscles immobilized by injury or illness. Less severe, but nevertheless damaging, atrophy results from the maintenance of certain postures for long periods of time, as in a factory job in which the arms are held in a forward position or in a desk job at which the worker sits with a "secretary slump." These are special cases in which certain muscles become atrophied because they are not being exercised to the same extent as other muscles of the body; specific exercises are needed for the unused muscles. All muscles will become atrophied to some extent when not worked regularly and, for this reason, regular systematic exercise is essential to maintenance of a desirable level of physical fitness.

Exercise is not a panacea for all ills, but together with good health habits, proper diet and a proper mental attitude, exercise can become a vital force in the life of an individual. Experience has proved that the well trained athlete is less susceptible to injury and recovers more rapidly than the athlete in poor condition. Exercise has increased the size of athletes' muscles, with an accompanying increase in the size of the tendons and an increase in the capillary system delivering blood to the muscle fibers. When added stress is placed upon the bone structure, there is a corresponding increase in the number of bone fibers so that the demands of power exertion can be met. The human mechanism is remarkable for its ability to adapt to various situations, and proper exercise can stimulate the various systems of the body to greater functional capacity.

One of the most important effects of exercise on the heart is that the increased number of capillary branches opens new avenues for delivering oxygen to the heart cells and also opens new routes for bypassing any injured or damaged area of the heart.

In addition to expanding the body's ability to adapt to the stimuli of internal and external forces, exercise can increase the efficiency of the body. The ability to perform life's daily tasks is an indication of the level of physical fitness that has been developed or acquired. Meeting such simple emergencies as shoveling out a snow drift, running to catch a bus and pushing a stalled car, situations in which sudden or explosive demands for energy are made upon the body, requires more than a minimal amount of fitness. The level of physical fitness necessary to perform the tasks of everyday living effectively and efficiently can be developed through exercise.

In participation in recreational sports, the well conditioned person is usually better coordinated, and he can enjoy the activity more fully because he has more stamina and better reflex action than the untrained person. Good physical condition is, in truth, a prerequisite for any sports participation if one is to enjoy himself to the fullest.

For the person who is not interested in sports participation, regular exercise provides an outlet from the relief of the tensions that are constantly with us and also promotes relaxation.

For those who have not taken any exercise of a serious nature at all, or at least not for a long period of time, the best advice possible is to proceed with caution. Many people with good intentions begin a program of exercise and then quit after the first day simply because they have overextended themselves and have consequently suffered great discomfort. This is a common error that can be avoided by using some restraint and following these few simple rules:

1. Spend more time warming up.
2. Before setting any standards for yourself, try each exercise a few times to get the feel of it.
3. Relax for a short time between exercises. Walk around if possible.
4. Increase your activity gradually until you reach the minimum standards for each exercise.
5. Stay with the MINIMUM standards until no undue stress is felt and there are no aftereffects.
6. Be regular in your exercise habits. Try to schedule your workout period at the same time each day, and accord it the same importance you would a business engagement.

PHYSICAL FITNESS

It has been stated previously that exercise is not a panacea for all ills. Likewise, there is no particular exercise or form of exercise which meets every physical need. Swimming has often been described as the most perfect form of exercise. The truth is that swimming has limitations. It does not, in itself, make you a better runner, high jumper, tennis player, etc. It does not improve your ability to do pull-ups, sit-ups and push-ups or to lift heavy objects. It is possible that just climbing out of a swimming pool accomplishes more in these respects. Today's better swimmers supplement their swimming activities with various forms of exercise or land training programs.

At this writing the latest fad to appeal to the fitness conscious public is jogging. Doctors, lawyers, teachers, housewives, students, professors and businessmen have all suddenly become heart conscious, and they are trying to rid their arteries of excess cholesterol, the number one suspect in atherosclerosis. As with most fads, immediate claims are being made as to the values of running, to the virtual exclusion of other forms of exercise. It is not our purpose here to downgrade swimming or running as forms of exercise or to disparage any claims of benefits to be derived from participation in these activities. Rather, it is our hope to establish their proper place in the total exercise program.

There are two areas of physical fitness which have become a major concern to the general public and the problems of both arise from lack of exercise.

In 1956 the findings of a team of specialists using the Kraus-Weber tests demonstrated that children in the United States did not rate as high on these simple tests (devised by the doctors to test their hospital patients) as did European children. Because of the publicity engendered by the results of these tests, the President of the United States considered it a serious enough problem to call a conference on Fitness of American Youth, which was held at the United States Naval Academy in Annapolis, Maryland, June 18 and 19, 1956. As a result of this conference, a President's Council on Physical Fitness was established by President Eisenhower. Presidents Kennedy and Johnson both deemed the problem of sufficient importance to continue and to improve upon the original program during their administrations.

Following the first conference, the American Association for Health, Physical Education and Recreation set up an elaborate testing program,* which was administered in test areas throughout the nation. These tests were designed to measure the elements of proficiency in the areas of running, jumping, throwing and climbing, as well as endurance. The test results indicated the poor physical condition of our schoolchildren, particularly in the areas of arm, chest and shoulder strength. The median scores on all tests were extremely low, which indicates that one half the children whose test scores fell below the median must have been in really poor physical condition. Scores on the running events did not appear to be so poor as those which measured the jumping, throwing and climbing ability of the youngsters.

The second problem primarily has involved the adult population and is commonly referred to as *heart failure.* Much of the research done in this area seems to indicate that the principal cause of the high incidence of heart attacks among United States males has been fatty degeneration of the inner coat of the arteries, a disease called atherosclerosis. Exercise has been advocated by prominent physicians and physical education people to overcome or to prevent further damage to the cardiac system.

---

*A.A.H.P.E.R. Youth Fitness Test Manual, Revised Edition. Washington, D.C., 1961.

Walking, cycling, swimming and jogging have all been recommended as good forms of exercise to aid in the prevention of heart problems and each is beneficial, but jogging has had the greatest appeal and, as a result, has received the greatest amount of publicity. "Run for Your Life" and "Jog for Health" clubs and groups have been forming all over the country and have enrolled thousands of members. At Yale University, during a five month period, more than 500 individuals participated in a "Run for Your Life" program, the ages of those taking part ranging from 18 to 65. Such extensive participation in jogging is encouraging to those who for so many years have been advocating participation in some form of exercise.

The enthusiasm for jogging or running should not obscure the fact that the benefits of this type of activity are limited for the achievement of body fitness. Cardiorespiratory efficiency is increased, but this is only one of the several components of total physical fitness.

The need for programs in the area of physical fitness has been emphasized continually by our Presidents and by national organizations concerned with the problem. The way of life for many people today, while not without mental stress, is definitely lacking situations which demand physical exertion. A regular program of exercise can be substituted for the daily chores and the rigors of life missing from today's environment. The exercises in this book are more than adequate to satisfy the body's need for strenuous activity. With this in mind, the following suggestions are made:

Medical examination

Before engaging in any exercise program to raise the level of physical fitness, each participant should have a thorough physical examination by a competent physician. Any physical limitations determined by the physician must be strictly observed. Adults beyond the age of 30 should have biennial examinations to determine their organic capabilities for the planned exercise program.

Regular exercise

A minimum of four workouts per week is recommended. Everyone, particularly those not in organized sports, should take regular exercise. Here are a few suggestions:
1. Do the Modern Daily Dozen, the Double Dozen, or the Big Ten every day (see Units II and III).
2. Exercise at the same time of day. Set aside that time as a necessary part of your life.
3. Participate with your family, a colleague or a friend. A specific date with someone will prevent your forgetting.

4. If you are an athlete, do the Modern Daily Dozen or the Double Dozen as a warm-up.
5. Do the exercises in addition to your recreational games and sports.

The exercises in the Modern Daily Dozen have been chosen to maintain or to develop different body areas and can be done with little or no equipment, in any attire, and, therefore, at any time of day or any season. The Modern Daily Dozen take 15 minutes to perform. Take the time, reap the benefits!

The exercises can be done on the floor, on a deck, in the classroom or in hallways. They require no special area. Naturally, if you do have special facilities and equipment, by all means use them, but remember to do the Modern Daily Dozen first. Supplement them with more elaborate types of exercise involving equipment, running or participation in competition. Give them a try for two weeks. See if your "tone," your well-being and your general enthusiasm for living have not increased tremendously. If possible, get into comfortable clothing in which to exercise and follow the activity with a shower.

PRINCIPLES OF WEIGHT REDUCTION

A calorie is defined as the amount of energy necessary to raise the temperature of one gram of water 1° centigrade. If the body needs only 1500 calories per day to perform all of the tasks required of it, and a person eats an amount of food supplying 2400 calories, there is then an excess of 900 calories which must be either burned up or stored as fat. If this same situation exists day after day, the weight of the body is going to increase unless sufficient work is performed to use up the excess calories.

Conversely, if the food intake amounts to 1500 calories and the work performed demands 2400 calories, there will be a deficit of 900 calories. Usually there are enough sugar and fat stored in the body to make up such a deficit temporarily, but a constant day-to-day deficit will result in severe weight loss.

If a person's present weight is ideal for his greatest efficiency, it would be to his advantage to maintain that weight level by consuming only enough food to perform his daily tasks, and no more. If the food intake remains constant and weight increases, there are two choices for the person to make: decrease the amount of food, or increase the amount of work.

The underweight person has a different problem. To gain weight he must increase the intake of high calorie foods to such an extent that his body will not burn up all the calories in work and exercise. Exercise is important to those who are underweight because it stimulates the appetite, which can then be satisfied by the consumption of large amounts of high calorie foods. Moreover, as muscles gain in strength as the result of exercise, they will add to the weight of the body.

Whether you are trying to lose or gain weight, it will be helpful to you to keep a constant check on your weight. It is important to take the measurement of your weight on the same scale, at the same time of day, and in the nude or wearing the same amount of clothing each time. Keep a chart with the days and dates projected, and possibly the weight you want to reach. This goal will be a constant reminder and will serve as an incentive. Another idea is to set your goals in the presence of a friend. Even a friendly bet that you will weigh "X" number of pounds at a certain date motivates action. The group therapy technique has been quite successful in helping people to stick to a diet and thus to accomplish the objectives of the plan involved. The values of sharing a problem with others in a similar situation and of committing oneself in the presence of others are obvious; the techniques could be applied with success to an exercise program as well as to dieting.

HEIGHT — WEIGHT — BODY BUILD STANDARDS (FOR BOTH SEXES)

A quick assessment of your physical status can be obtained by referring to the accompanying height and weight table, which takes into consideration your body build and your sex.

Great emphasis has been given to body weight. Medical authorities have attributed many health problems and diseases to overweight. Excessive overweight or underweight can be considered to be 15 per cent deviation from the norm for your height and body build.

It has been previously stated that weight can be influenced and controlled through exercise. However, there are other factors which contribute to the weight problem, such as heredity, metabolic rate and overeating. These are complex considerations and are beyond the scope of this discussion.

In four weeks' time, through a moderate change in the quality and the quantity of food intake, your weight can be increased or decreased. Exercise as presented here will assist you with your weight problem and will give tonus (firmness) to your body. Diet and exercise in moderation and do not become discouraged during the first two-week period. Since your weight can fluctuate daily, give it your attention over a prolonged period of time.

If you are trying to lose weight, a little psychological trick is to be discerning about your diet for six days of the week so that on the

Table 1. Desirable Weights for Men and Women[*]
Weight in Pounds According to Frame (In Indoor Clothing)

Men

Height With Shoes on (1-inch heels)	Small Frame	Medium Frame	Large Frame
5′ 2″	112-120	118-129	126-141
5′ 3″	115-123	121-133	129-144
5′ 4″	118-126	124-136	132-148
5′ 5″	121-129	127-139	135-152
5′ 6″	124-133	130-143	138-156
5′ 7″	128-137	134-147	142-161
5′ 8″	132-141	138-152	147-166
5′ 9″	136-145	142-156	151-170
5′10″	140-150	146-160	155-174
5′11″	144-154	150-165	159-179
6′ 0″	148-158	154-170	164-186
6′ 1″	152-162	158-175	168-189
6′ 2″	156-167	162-180	173-194
6′ 3″	160-171	167-185	178-199
6′ 4″	164-175	172-190	182-204

Women

Height With Shoes on (2-inch heels)	Small Frame	Medium Frame	Large Frame
4′10″	92- 98	96-107	104-119
4′11″	94-101	98-110	106-122
5′ 0″	96-104	101-113	109-125
5′ 1″	99-107	104-116	112-128
5′ 2″	102-110	107-119	115-131
5′ 3″	105-113	110-122	118-134
5′ 4″	108-116	113-126	121-138
5′ 5″	111-119	116-130	125-142
5′ 6″	114-123	120-135	129-146
5′ 7″	118-127	124-139	133-150
5′ 8″	122-131	128-143	137-154
5′ 9″	126-135	132-147	141-158
5′10″	130-140	136-151	145-163
5′11″	134-144	140-155	149-168
6′ 0″	138-148	144-159	153-173

[*]Metropolitan Life Insurance Company.

seventh day you can go "off" your plan and eat almost anything. If you check your weight and compare it with your previous record, you will probably find that your seventh day fling has not affected your weight.

Your weight can be controlled effectively by a good exercise program. According to Jean Mayer, D.S.C., of Harvard University: "It has been demonstrated mathematically that one half hour of proper exercise each day could keep off or take off as much as 26 pounds a year."

There are some excellent general guidelines for the overweight individual which have been drawn from the results of experimental research studies and actuary norms coupled with good judgment. Here are a few:

A common belief is that there is a serious danger in being overweight. This is true only if you are excessively overweight or more than 15 per cent above or below the average weight for persons of your height, sex and build.

A desirable weight at 25 is considered to be your desirable weight throughout the rest of your life.

Check yourself against the chart and keep a daily log of your weight.

Stop eating as soon as you go over your daily calorie quota.

Keep to a six-day program of limited calorie intake.

Get dressed and go out socially at least once a week. This will help you to be conscious of yourself, and your pride oftentimes will stimulate you into doing something about your appearance.

UNIT II

HOW TO BEGIN
CIRCUIT TRAINING
THE FIRST DOZEN
AN EVALUATION
THE SECOND DOZEN

HOW TO BEGIN

There are two complete sets of 12 exercises each on the following pages. The first 12 exercises are called the Modern Daily Dozen. The name is derived from the title, The Daily Dozen, given to a set of exercises published many years ago by Walter Camp, a former Yale football coach and author of 16 books, perhaps most widely known for his weekly column in Colliers magazine in which were published his All-American selections of football players from the years 1891 to 1925. At the time of the appearance of the Daily Dozen in print (incidentally, they proved very popular) he introduced the dozen exercises with these remarks: "The investment called for is ten minutes of your time and a little common sense. The returns on this investment are longer life, increased happiness, and greater business efficiency. The vigor of good health is the biggest single factor in success. It is the dynamo that supplies the motive power of the brains." Today, professional physical educators might hedge on the longer life claims of Mr. Camp, but most would heartily endorse his other observations. The Modern Daily Dozen offers you an opportunity to make the investment and reap the benefits of which he spoke.

The second set consists of 12 more exercises that provide more difficulty and challenge than the first set. They may be incorporated as single items or as a whole set with the first dozen exercises. The two sets together are known as The Double Dozen.

Begin with the Modern Daily Dozen, and after trying each exercise for difficulty, allot a specific amount of time for it. The warm-up is the first exercise and it is very important. Devote four minutes to this first exercise and the suggested variations given. After the warm-up do the next 11 exercises, devoting exactly 1 minute to each one. Set your own pace, preferably at a slow rate of speed the first time.

The pace can be increased some on each following day. The purpose of the time element is to increase the number of repetitions for each exercise in the minute allotted, thereby increasing the stress put upon the body. The total time for the first dozen exercises done in the above manner will be 15 minutes, the *minimum* daily amount of time recommended by the President's Council on Physical Fitness.

Once the 15-minute session of exercise becomes routine, the next step in the process is to increase the time you devote to each exercise. For example, perform the warm-up 4½ minutes and each of the following exercises 1 minute and 15 seconds.

When you have done the first dozen exercises long enough to feel that you would like some variation in the routine, read "An Evaluation" (page 28) and comments on the Second Dozen (page 28). Follow the same procedure with the second set of exercises if you are going to use them as a unit, testing your ability to do them properly. If you do not wish to use them as an entire unit at first, add the second set of exercises to the first dozen one by one.

CIRCUIT TRAINING

In the previous routine you have used the Daily Dozen and The Double Dozen, devoting a specific amount of time to each exercise. A form of circuit training can be developed using these exercises. For each exercise, three circuits are established (labeled first, second and third). A goal is determined for each of the circuits consisting of a set number of repetitions for each exercise. Each circuit consists of three rounds.

The circuit for the least difficult number of repetitions is called the "first circuit." This circuit is for beginners and all others who are not in top condition. Begin with this circuit. You can move on to a more difficult one later. Next in order of difficulty is the "second circuit" which has been set up for those who are in good physical condition. For the top athlete the "third circuit" has been set up with the greatest number of repetitions. You will see three circles, each with different numbers, beside each exercise, on pages 15 to 41.

If you find that the first circuit is too difficult for you, cut down on the number of repetitions and work slowly. *Each circuit should be done three times without pause.* Before you move on to the second circuit, be sure that you can do the first one to the peak of your capacity. Do not attempt to do the third circuit until the second one can be done efficiently, and you are sure that you cannot improve further on the time that it takes you to complete three rounds.

One of the reasons for using circuit training as a means of improving your physical attributes is the personal factor of self improve-

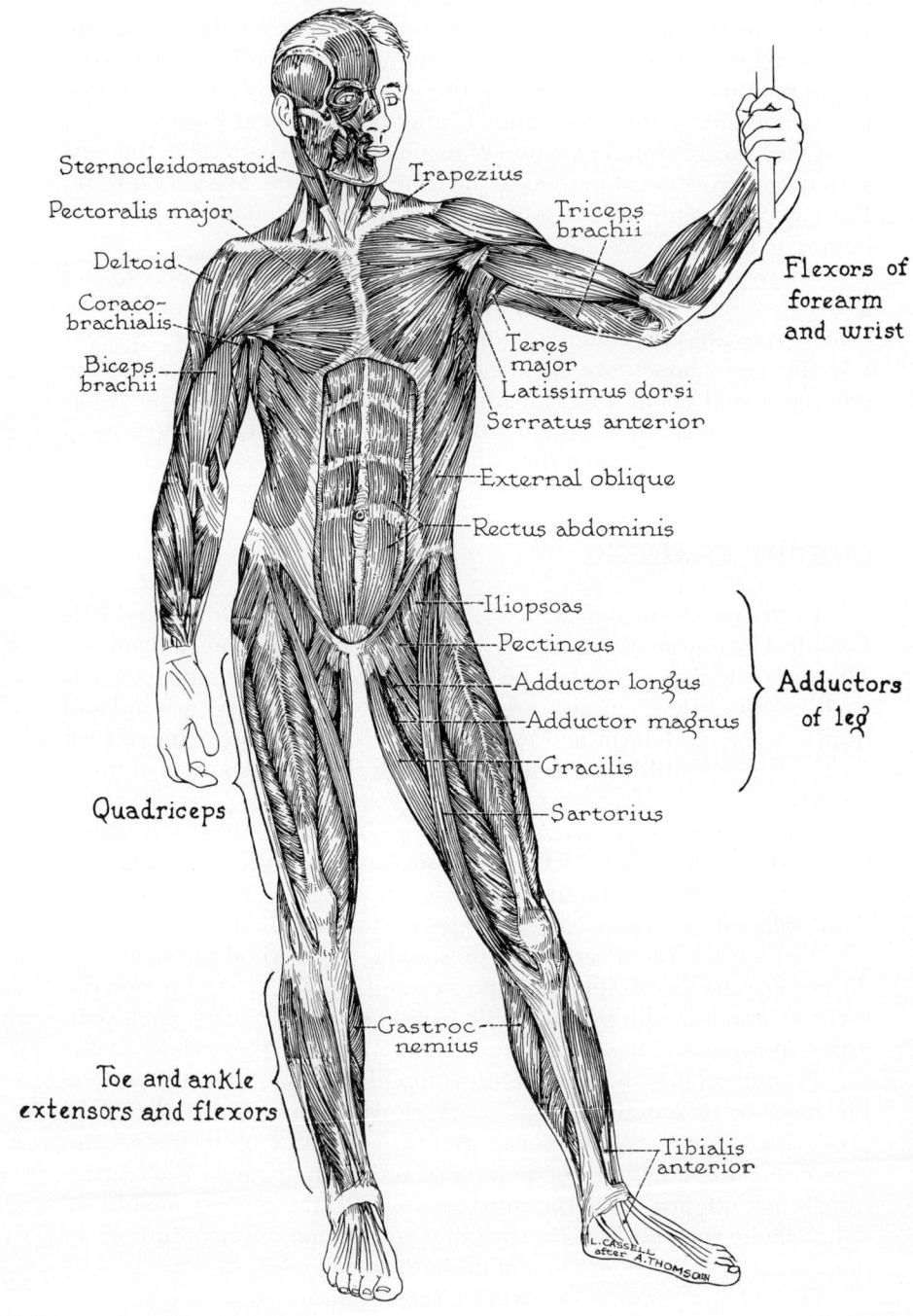

BODY CONDITIONING FOR COLLEGE MEN 13

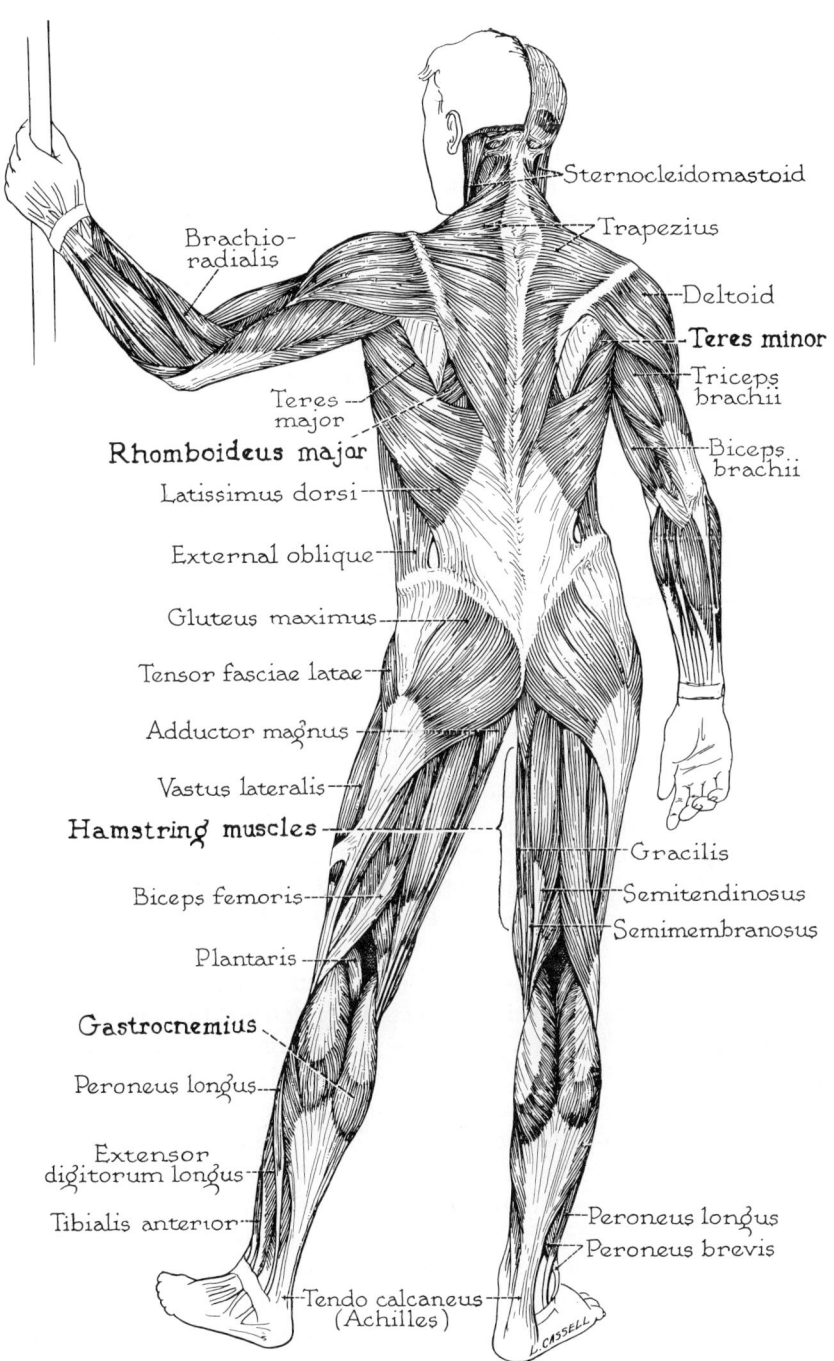

ment. You will be working against yourself trying to better each previous effort before moving on to the next stage of difficulty. Be honest in your attempts to perform each individual exercise. Do not cut corners. Daily use of the first circuit is better than trying the second circuit once or twice a week.

A sample workout is given here to clarify the procedure. In the first circle next to the illustration of the first exercise, Jumping Jacks, (page 15) are the numbers 15-20. This means to repeat the exercise 15 to 20 times. Below the Jumping Jack exercises are listed eight more warm-up exercises. Do each one of these 15 to 20 times. This should take about four minutes. The second exercise is called the Twister, and in the first circle it is suggested that this exercise be done ten times on each side. (If the number of repetitions seems to be too low, remember that you will be repeating the exercise again in the second and third rounds.) Follow the directions given and then do the exercise the prescribed number of times.

The third exercise is Push-ups, and the prescribed number of times is eight in the first circle.

The fourth exercise is Rise and Shine, and the first circle indicates that you are going to sit up and touch your toes ten times.

Follow this procedure through the remainder of the first 12 exercises. Do exercise number 5, the Leg Stretcher, five times. Exercise number 6, Curls, is done ten times. Exercise number 7 is a change of pace exercise, and you can set your own number of repetitions if 25 times will be too many or too few.

Exercise number 8 is called Chop Chop, and is performed slowly ten times. Exercise number 9 is done 15 times; number 10 is done ten times; number 11 is done six times, and number 12, Trunk Twist Neck Press, is done ten times on each side. This completes one round of the circuit. Proper procedure, under ideal conditions, is to immediately repeat these 12 exercises a second time, and then again a third time. Let your condition be your guide as to how much you can do the first day. Caution is recommended for the beginner. For anyone finding it too easy, increase the dosage by moving up to the second circuit. However, try to do three rounds of the first circuit efficiently and properly before attempting the second circuit. When the second circuit can be done three times efficiently, then attempt the third circuit.

It should be remembered that each person may vary either ahead or below his age category. The idea is to find out by trial and error in doing the circuit how many repetitions of each exercise can be done within comfortable limits and then try to cut down the time it takes to do it. As time goes on, you will know the exercises and only spot checks will be necessary.

THE FIRST DOZEN

Jumping Jacks

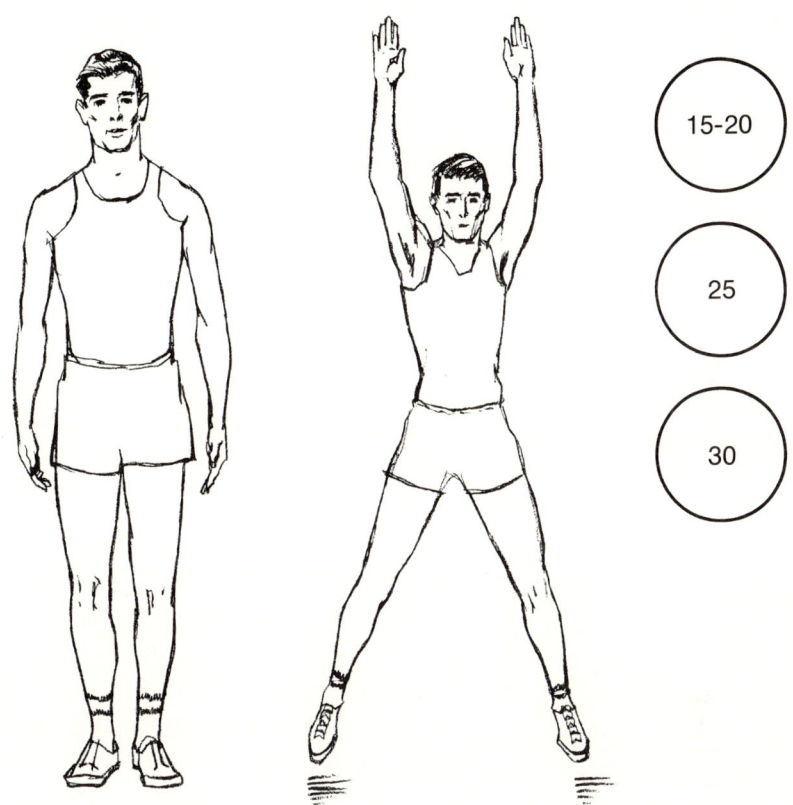

Purpose: To increase the circulation and get the body "warmed up." When the body is thoroughly "heated," heavier exercise can be performed without undue strain.

Position: Stand with feet slightly apart, arms at sides.

Exercise: Jump, feet apart, hands overhead, on the count of one. Return to position on the count of two. Repeat.

Suggestions: Bounce on the balls of the feet, with the heels slightly off the ground or floor. Begin slowly and gradually increase the tempo.

Other warm-up exercises

1. Place feet together. Hop up and down in place, landing on the balls of the feet. Hands can be placed on hips or behind the neck.
2. Same as above. Hop forward and back.
3. Same as above. Hop side to side.
4. Hop on left foot, repeat on right foot.
5. Jump stride and then cross feet instead of bringing them together.
6. Walk stride. Alternate striding forward and back. Swing arms alternately.
7. Goose step and increase tempo.
8. Jog in place.

The Twister

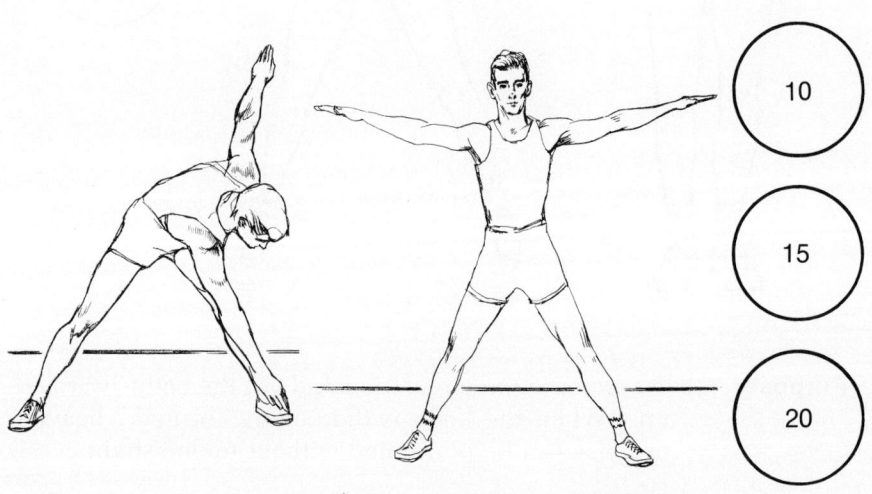

Purpose: To activate the erector spinae muscles of the lower back as well as the upper arm and back muscles; to stretch the hamstring muscles in the backs of the legs; to exercise the lateral trunk muscles.

Position: Stand, feet wide apart, arms held at sides horizontally.

Exercise: Bend forward at the waist and, at the same time, twist the trunk, touching the right hand to the left foot and swinging the left hand high to a vertical position on the count of one. Return to position on the count of two. Alternate to the other side on counts three and four. Repeat.

Suggestions: For a more violent exercise, the above may be performed with the trunk bent from the waist as the starting position, with the arms stretched sideward. A vigorous alternate twist and toe touch is then done with a one-two count.

Push-ups

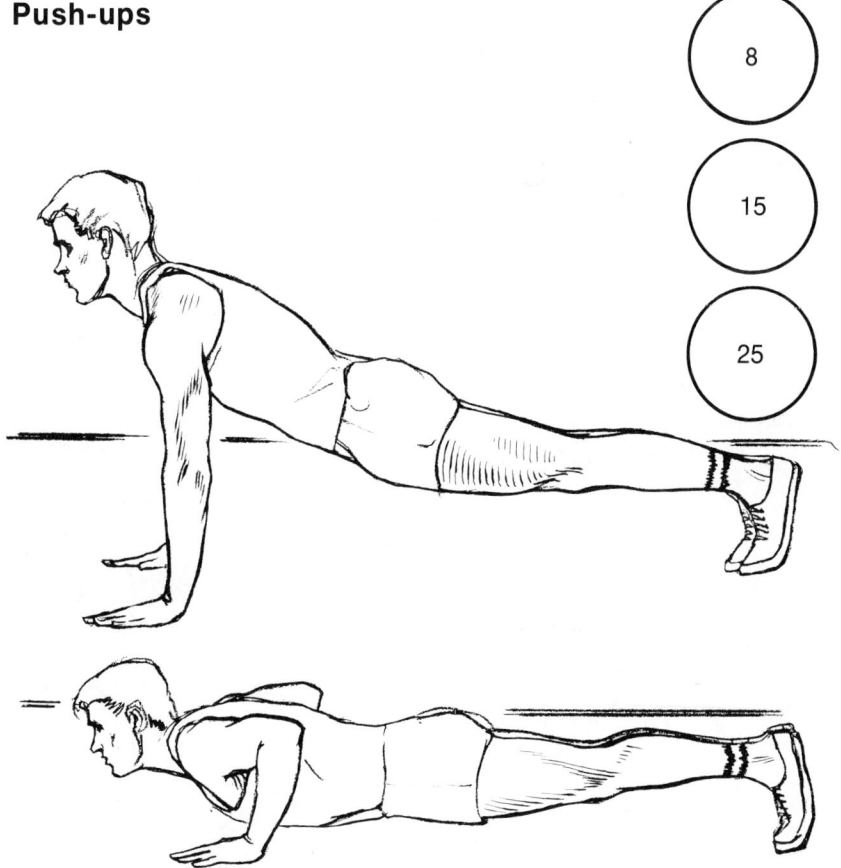

Purpose: To develop the muscles of the chest (pectoralis), the forward part of the deltoid muscle located in the shoulder and the triceps muscle located at the back of the upper arm. The greatest emphasis is on the triceps.

Position: Assume a front leaning rest position with the body in a straight line from the shoulders to the heels. Rest on the toes and hands with the arms straight.

Exercise: On the count of one, bend the elbows until the chest touches the floor. Without changing body alignment, push up again to a front leaning rest on the count of two.

Suggestions: This is a difficult exercise if done correctly. Variations are possible to make the exercise easier without changing body position, such as resting on the knees and toes instead of toes alone, or placing the hands on a chair or table and stepping back far enough so that the legs and trunk are extended. The push up movement is then performed as described above.

If it is desirable to make the exercise more vigorous, begin as in the original position and on the count of two, push up and clap hands, or on the count of two, push up and touch the chest with the fingertips.

Rise and Shine (Sit-ups)

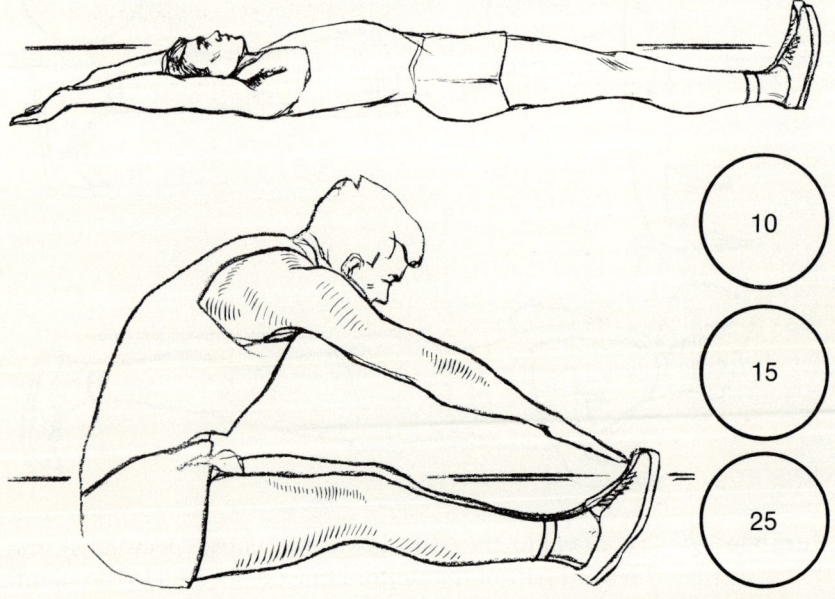

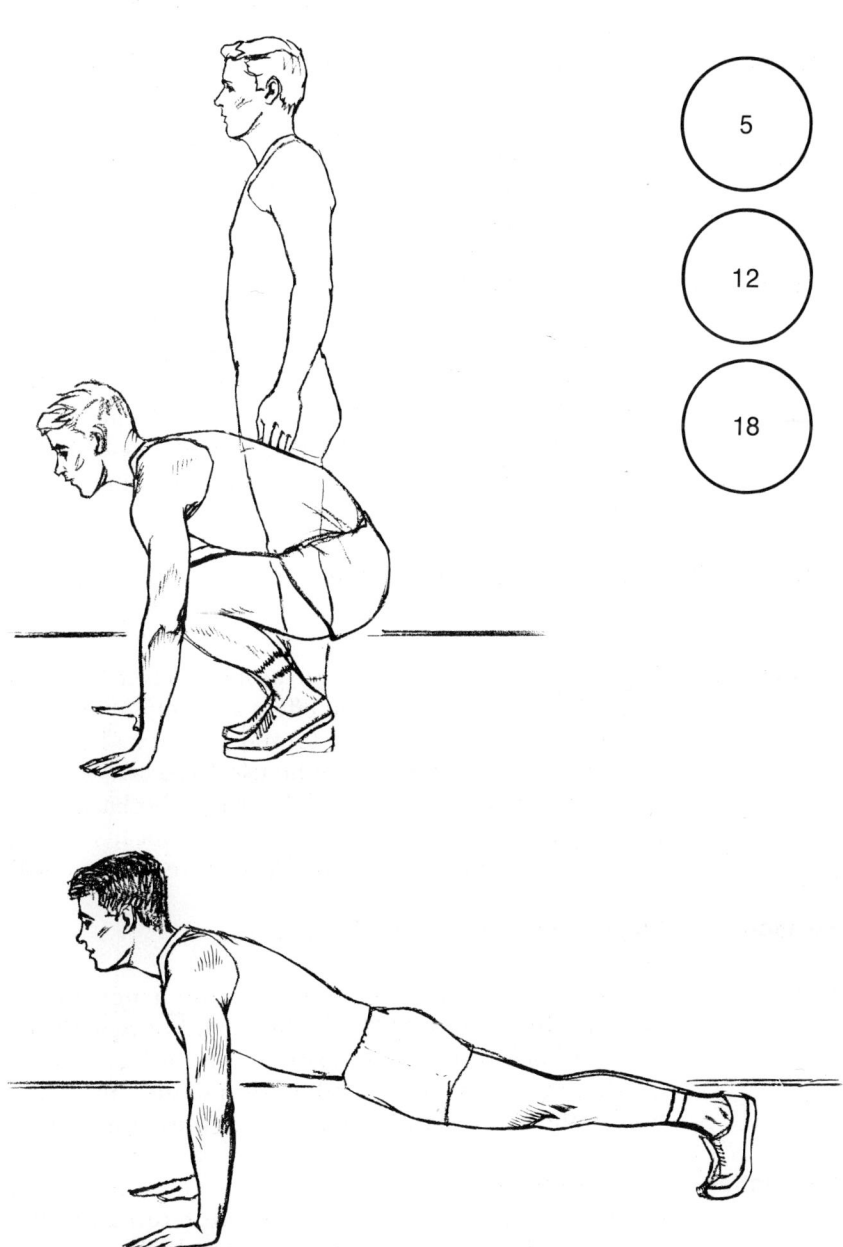

Purpose: To develop the abdominal and hip flexor muscles. This exercise with legs straight places the emphasis on the hip flexor group, while the bent knee position places the emphasis on the abdominal group.

Position: Lie on back with arms extended overhead, feet apart, and knees slightly bent.

Exercise: Sit up and bend forward reaching to toes or beyond with hands. Return to position. Use four counts; go up on one-two and back on three-four.

Suggestions: For those who wish to make the exercise less taxing, begin by raising the arms with a vigorous swing up toward the toes. If the feet are anchored between or under an immovable object the exercise is also easier. If the desire is to make the work more strenuous, go through the exercise slowly. If the hands are held behind the neck, the exercise is also more strenuous.

The Leg Stretcher (Squat Thrusts)

Purpose: This exercise serves many purposes since it involves three different positions and offers a variety of options. It can also be used as a test for measuring agility and, if done for a long period, can be used as a test of stamina. The extensor muscles of the arms, the back muscles along the spine and the leg extensors located in the buttock region and the back of the legs are all exercised.

Position: Stand with arms at sides, feet apart.

Exercise: Bend to a squat position and place the hands on the floor on the count of one. On the count of two, thrust the feet back so that the position of front leaning rest (push-up position) is reached. Return to the squat position on the count of three. Stand up on the count of four.

Suggestions: For variety, add a push-up when the legs are in the extended position. When the legs are returned to the squat position, instead of standing up, do the duck-up exercise, one of the second dozen, before standing up.

Curls

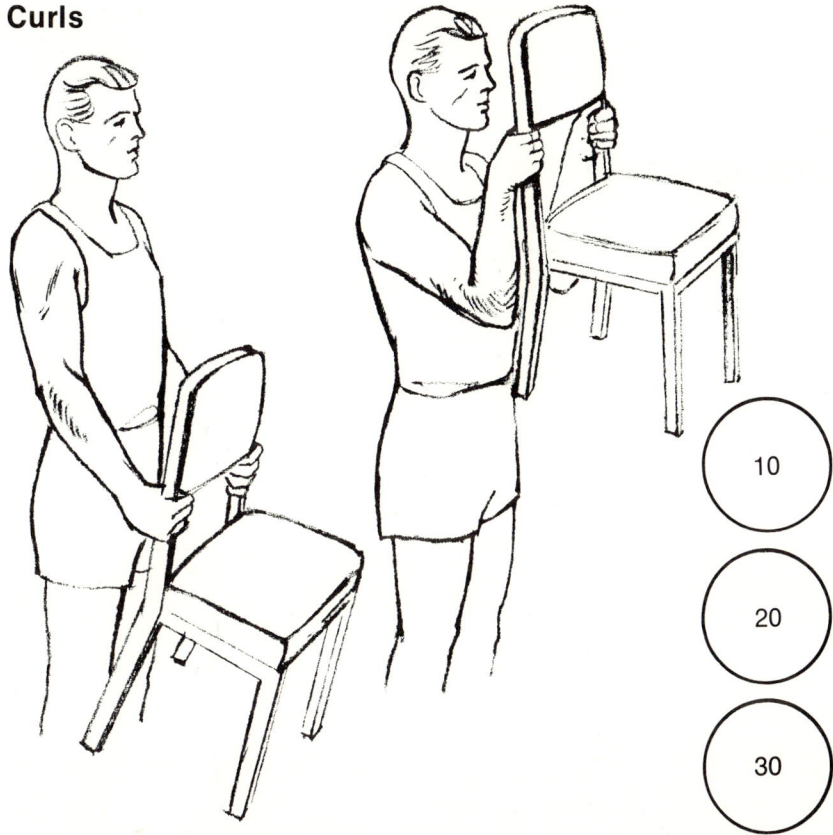

Purpose: To develop the flexor muscles of the elbow which raise the hand to the shoulder and are very important for pull ups, yet are usually neglected in most exercise programs which do not have pulley weights or regular barbells. The heavier the object raised, the greater the development of these muscles.

Position: Stand with feet slightly apart and hold an object in hands at hip level. Object should be fairly heavy, such as a chair or sandbag.

Exercise: Raise the chair or object to chest level on count of one and return to position on count of two.

Suggestions: This is an exercise in which equipment is useful, such as the chair suggested above. However, isometric exercise can be used to good advantage in this instance. If a person is seated at a desk, he can place his hands palms up under the desk while in sitting position and lift up. This can be done with the elbow joint flexed in varied positions.

Jogging in Place

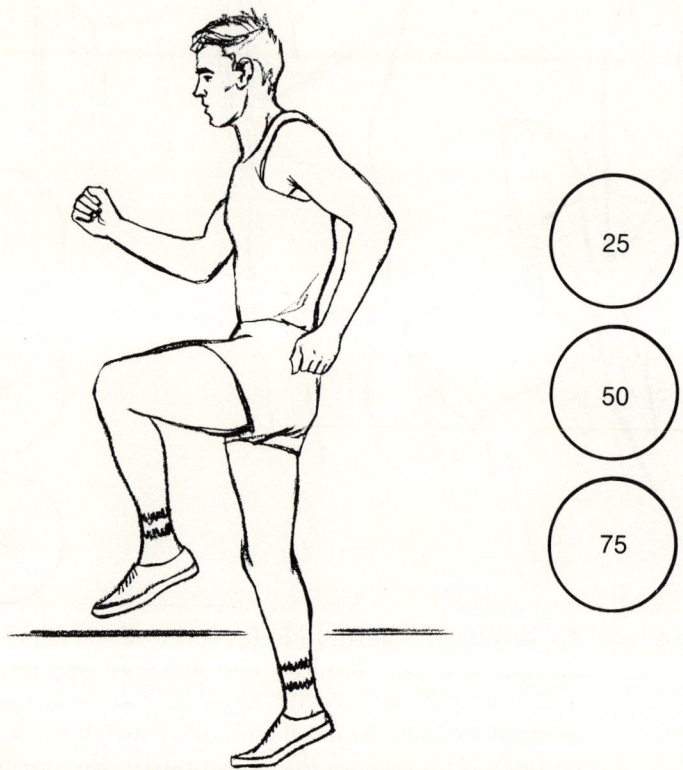

Purpose: To develop cardiorespiratory endurance. Jogging offers variation to the routine and increases the blood circulation. Running, of course, is one of the best forms of exercise for building stamina.

Position: Stand with arms at sides.

Exercise: A jog is a slow run or trot. In this instance, it is done without moving from the same position on the floor or ground. The movement should begin slowly and increase gradually until the arms are being pumped vigorously upward with elbows bent and fists partly clenched. The knees should be brought up high and should almost reach the chest.

Suggestions: Try to simulate the natural movement of running as much as possible. Build up to peaks, slow down gradually and then increase the tempo again.

Chop Chop (Cross Arms and Legs)

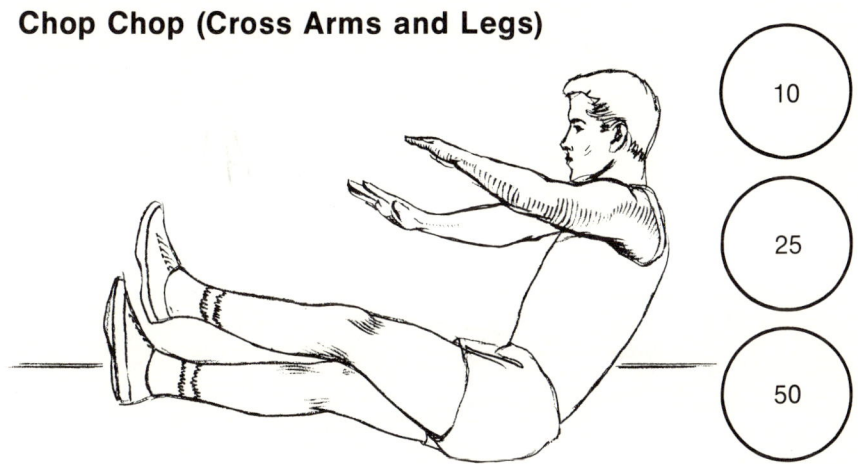

Purpose: To exercise the muscles located in the lower abdominal and hip area, including the rectus abdominis muscle, the flexor muscles of the thigh and the abductor and adductor muscles of the leg. Smaller muscles in the shoulder and chest region are also involved.

Position: Sit with arms at forward horizontal position, feet raised a few inches off the floor. Each person must find his or her own balance position by leaning back and raising both legs at the same time.

Exercise: Cross hands and feet alternately without allowing the feet to touch the floor. The action should be rapid movement of both arms and legs without too much spread of either one. Arms and legs are extended throughout the exercise.

Suggestions: First practice balancing on the buttocks and the end of the spine. It is good practice to lean back with the head and trunk before lifting the feet from the floor. Begin with slow movements and gradually increase the speed.

Trunk Dips

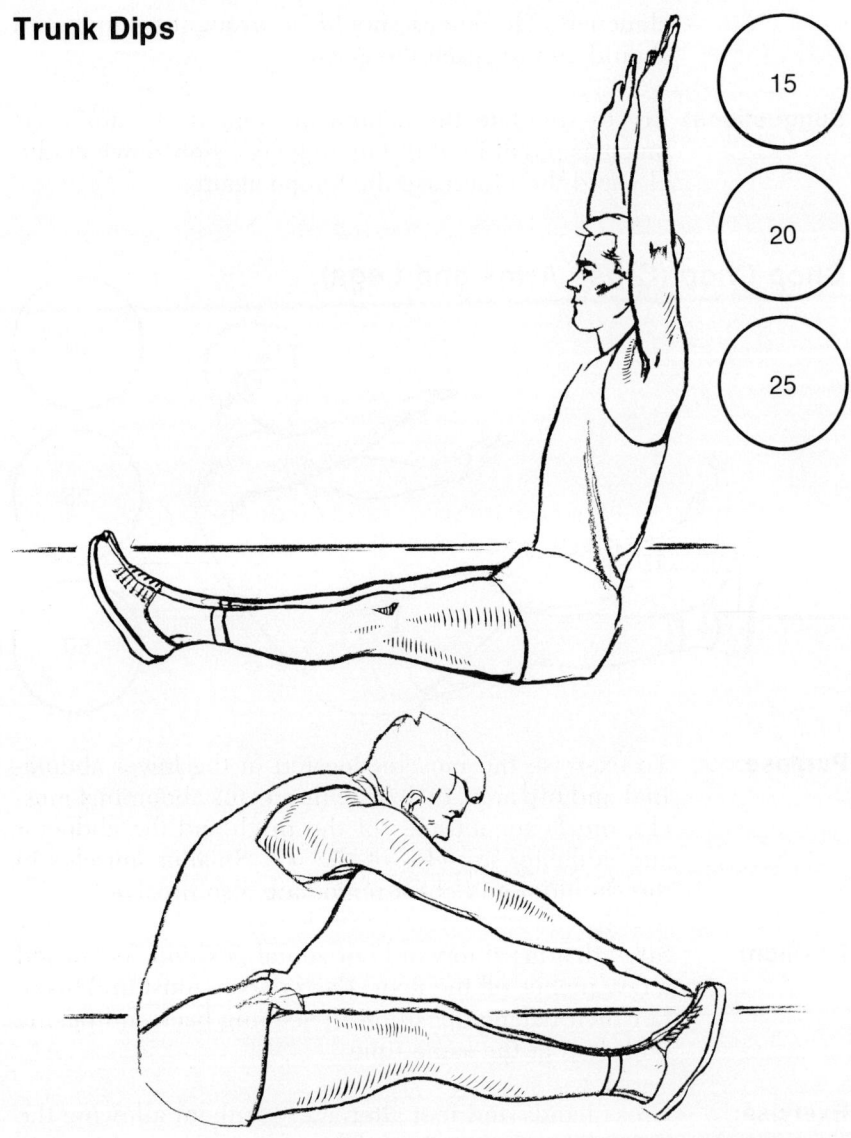

Purpose: To stretch the lower back muscles and the hamstring muscles of the legs. Stretching in itself is beneficial for increasing flexibility.

Position: Sit with legs extended, feet slightly apart, the trunk and head erect and the arms extended vertically overhead.

Exercise: On the count of one, bend forward and try to touch the hands to toes without lowering the arms before the head and trunk. On counts of two and three, stretch forward a little more on each count. On the count of four, return to the original position.

Suggestions: This exercise, if done with four counts as above, can be made less demanding with four rest counts between each movement of the exercise. In this way, more emphasis can be made on the stretch up before starting to bend forward, and the pattern of muscular contraction and relaxation can be maintained.

Pig-a-Back

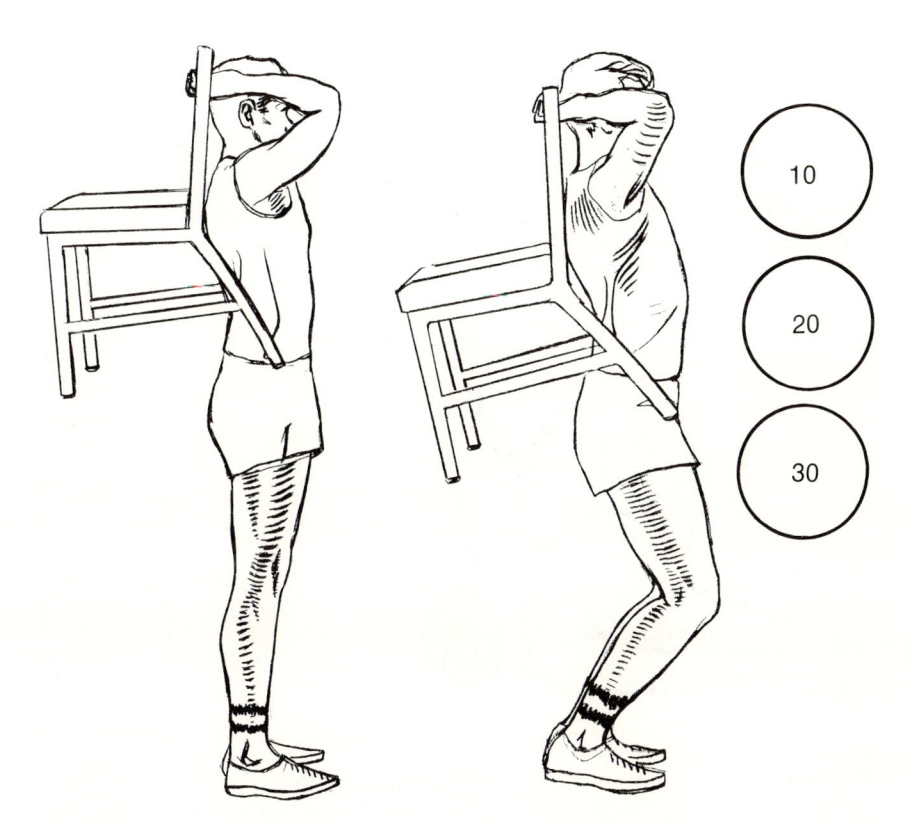

Purpose: To strengthen the knee extensor (quadriceps) and hip extensor (gluteus maximus) muscles.

Position: Stand with feet spread 12 to 16 inches apart. Hold a chair or any object of similar weight on or in back of the shoulders.

Exercise: Bend the knees to a one-half squat position on the count of one and return to position on the count of two.

Suggestions: Try to keep the trunk fairly erect and the feet flat at all times. Do not bend the knees more than halfway. In order to increase the work in this exercise, the amount of weight must be increased or the number of repetitions increased.

Liver Squeezer (Knee Raising to Chest)

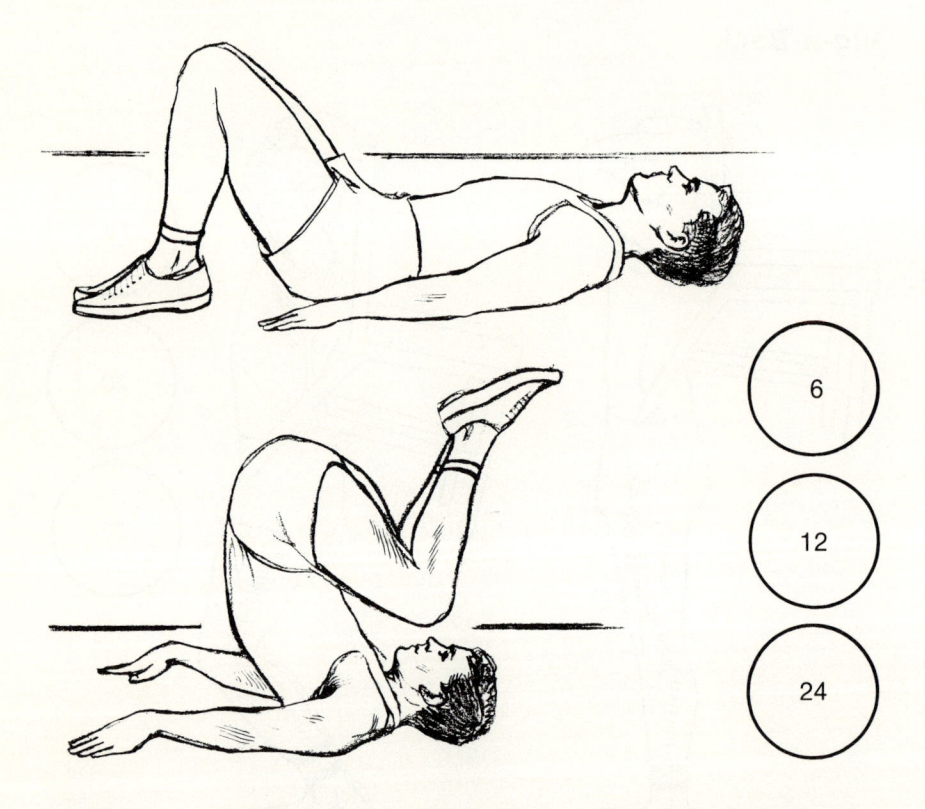

6

12

24

Purpose: To develop the abdominal muscles (rectus abdominis). There are many other muscles involved, including the knee flexors, the arm extensors and the muscles of the upper back and shoulders.

Position: Lie on the back with the knees bent and the heels close to the buttocks. Keep the arms extended at the sides with the hands at hip level.

Exercise: Begin with the heels off the floor and raise the knees up to the chest, bringing the hips up high overhead. It is most important that the heels be kept in tight against the buttocks all during the exercise. Use four counts; bring the knees up on one, hold on two and three, and down on four.

Suggestions: If the work is too difficult to do correctly at the beginning, change the position by extending the legs and return the legs to the extended position each time. This would require four counts as above, but would be feet to buttocks and knees to chest on the count of one, hold on two and extend the legs to position on three and four.

Trunk Twist Neck Press

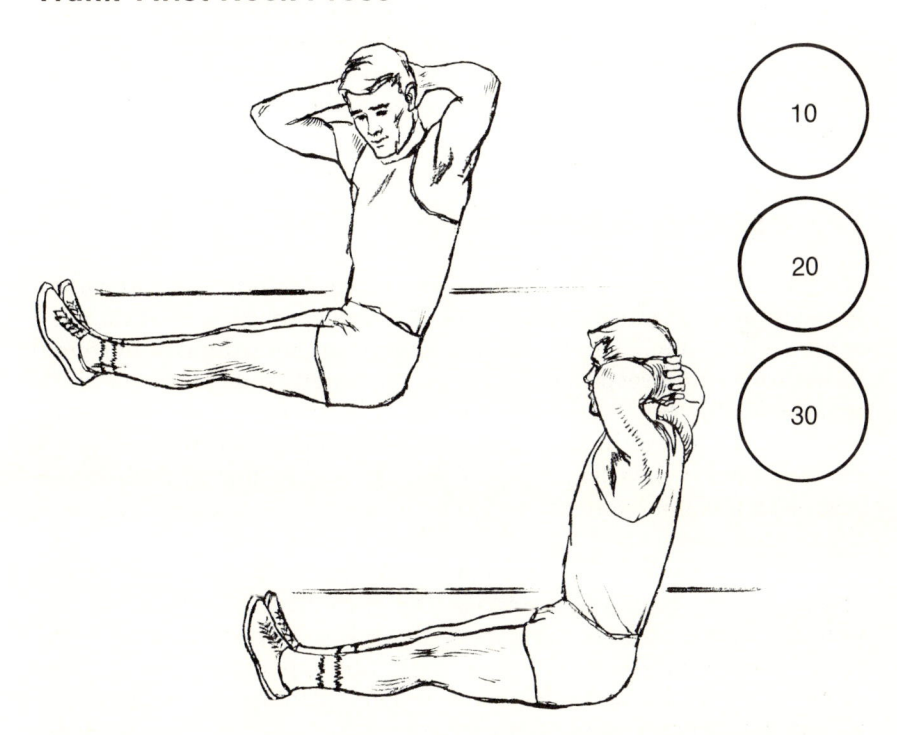

10

20

30

Purpose: To strengthen the external and internal oblique (lateral trunk) muscles. The neck press exercises the rhomboid and trapezius muscles in the upper back, the wrist flexors and the triceps in the back of the arm, which normally extend the elbow joint.

Position: Sit with the legs extended, hands behind the head and neck, body erect and the elbows well back.

Exercise: Twist the trunk to the left on the count of one and all the way around to the right on the count of two. Alternate twisting left and right without pause. At the same time, draw the chin in slightly and press the back of the head backward against the hands.

AN EVALUATION

It is time to appraise the effort you have expended and to take stock of your physical condition. Do these 12 exercises show that you are in worse shape than you had suspected? Or are you better? If these first 12 exercises are too difficult, use the easier variations suggested and proceed more slowly. If they have proved to be just right, continue until you can perform all of them without having to refer to the book. Increase the amount of exercise slightly as you go along. If there is no difficulty at this point and all the exercises can be done properly without reference to the book, begin adding more exercises from the second dozen.

THE SECOND DOZEN

The 12 exercises already presented have included a good variety of positions and movements which are necessary for a well-rounded exercise program. Included in this first group are exercises designed to improve cardiorespiratory efficiency, strength and the power of the muscles of the legs, arms and shoulders, abdomen, back and lateral muscles of the trunk. Also included are movements to assist in increasing agility and flexibility. Taken as a unit, this is probably as complete a set of exercises as is necessary for your needs. Why then a second dozen?

There are many good reasons for adding a second set of movements to one's program of activity. It is done here specifically to provide the opportunity to emphasize the action in certain areas of the body where definite weaknesses exist. Young people probably need more work on the arms, legs and abdominal muscles, while adults should concentrate more on the muscles which are involved in movement in the middle third of the body. There are also movements in the second dozen which help considerably to improve flexibility. Since variety is considered by many to be the spice of life, here variety is provided to spice up your exercise program.

This second group of 12 exercises can be taken in whole or in part, depending on your needs. For those who are already in good physical condition, they can be added gradually to the first dozen, or both units can be combined and the Double Dozen used as one unit. This combination should meet the demands of the most ardent exercise fan.

When additional exercises are combined with the first unit, it is advisable to experiment in the same manner as prescribed with the first group. It is suggested that each exercise be tried only a few times to get the feel of it before incorporating it in your regular program.

Some of the exercises in this second group are quite difficult to do the first time and it may be advisable to do them first only partially. Included in the group of hard-to-perform exercises are the Jack-knife, Hip Dips, Frustrator, Bridge Up, Grinder and Double Trouble. Follow the suggestions given with each of these movements if easier action is necessary. Suggestions are also made in some instances for increasing the work load.

Hopping

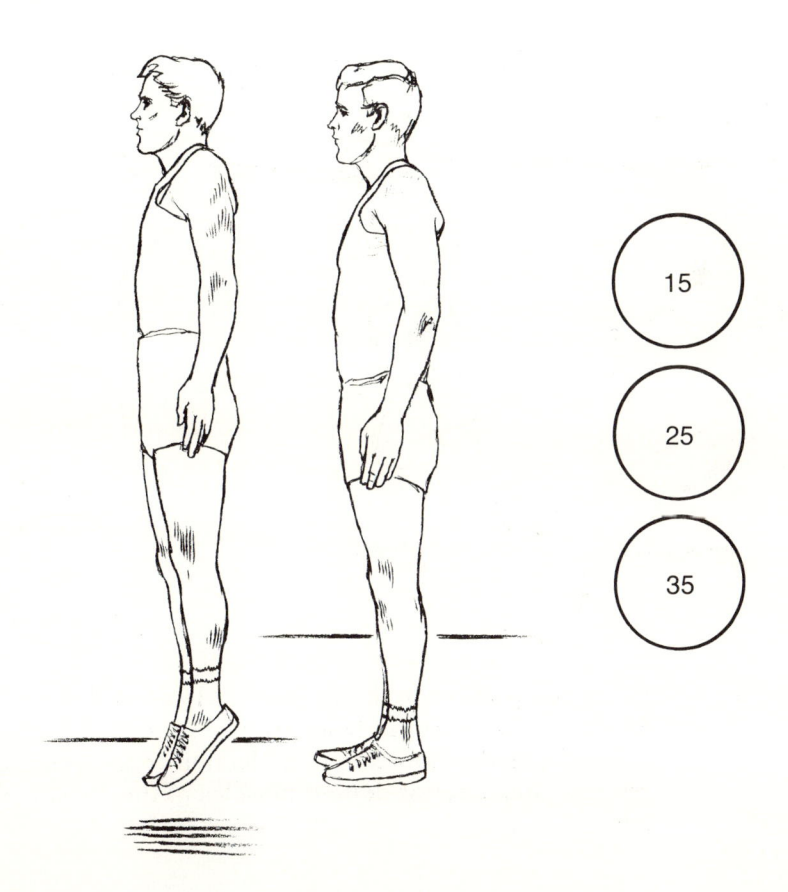

Purpose: To develop the muscles which extend the ankle (gastrocnemius and soleus) and the knee (quadriceps group). Used along with Jumping Jacks and Jogging, it helps to provide an excellent warm-up movement.

Position: Stand with feet slightly apart and arms at sides.

Exercise: Hop up and down on balls of the feet. Try to push up just enough so that the toes just clear the floor with the ankle joint fully extended. Vary this exercise by hopping forward and back and also left to right.

Suggestions: Hopping provides movement that changes the tempo of a routine. The exercise can be made more strenuous by carrying objects on the shoulders which add weight and increase the work load.

The Jack-knife

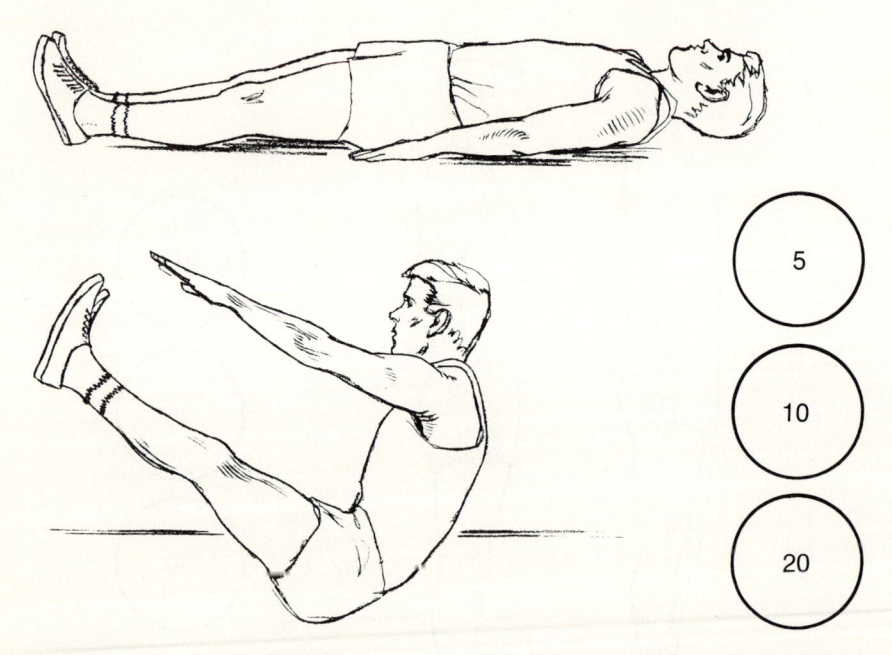

5

10

20

Purpose: To develop the hip flexor and abdominal muscles. Swinging the arms horizontally from the side to the forward position (horizontal adduction) exercises the pectoral and anterior deltoid muscles of the chest and arms.

Position: Lie on the back with legs straight, ankles extended, feet slightly apart and arms on the floor close to the sides of the body.

Exercise: Raise the feet off the floor and at the same time sit up partway and touch the toes with the fingertips, all on the count of one. Return to the supine position on two. If slower movement is desirable, use two counts to raise up, and two counts to return to position.

Suggestions: For the purpose of coordinating this movement, begin with the hands next to the hips; as the head is raised from the floor, keep the fingers close to the thighs and reach forward toward the toes. Gradually raise the shoulders and back off the floor as the hands are moved forward and the legs raised. After a few experimental tries, the arms can gradually be moved sideward until the best position is reached for ease of movement. Persons with heavy legs will find this exercise difficult to master, but a slight bend of the knees will facilitate the movement. The exercise can be made more difficult by performing the movements slowly. Change from a two count to a four count tempo to do this.

Hip Dips

Purpose: To develop the hip abductors.

Position: Side at leaning rest. This position is easily taken by first sitting on the side of the left hip with legs extended. The left foot is kept in front of the right and the left hand serves as a base. The base hand is placed on the floor directly under the left shoulder. The right hand can be kept on the hip or, for a better position, behind the neck. The hips are raised up from the floor so that the body is in a straight line from the shoulder to the ankle. This is the side leaning rest position.

Exercise: From the above position, drop the left hip down toward the floor on the count of one and return to position on the count of two.

Suggestions: If the movement is too difficult to do, a change in the starting position might be of help. Begin in the side sitting position instead of side leaning and build up to the proper method slowly. Keep the legs extended.

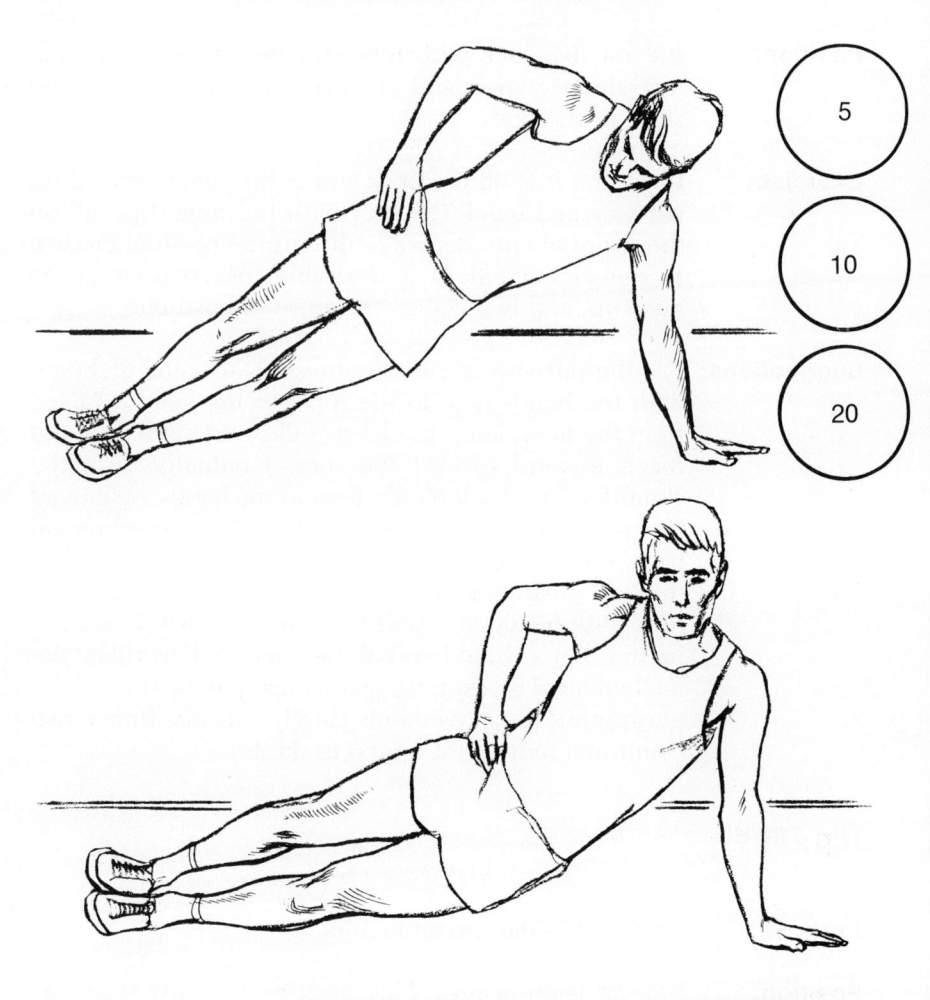

The Hurdle

Purpose: To stretch the hamstring muscles of the legs.

Position: Sit in a hurdle position as follows: Sit down with both legs extended. Turn the great toe of the left foot toward the right foot and at the same time draw the heel of the left foot back toward the left hip. If possible, try to form a right angle, with the right leg straight forward and the left leg out to the side with the knee bent.

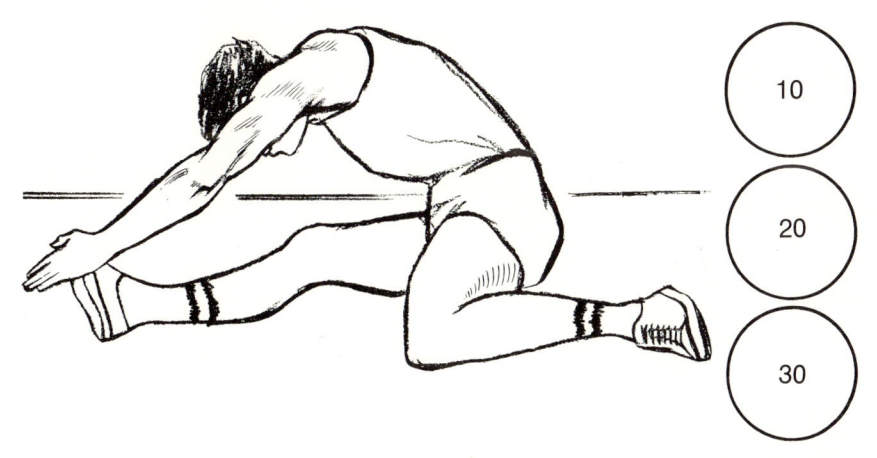

Exercise: Grasp the right knee or the right foot with both hands and bend the trunk as far forward as possible. Increase the movement a little more by pulling against the right leg. This is a two count exercise, but if the movement is done rapidly, count only the number of times the the trunk goes forward. Repeat to the opposite side.

Suggestions: Depending upon the amount of flexibility present, this exercise can be simple or extremely difficult. If you find it almost impossible to do, ease up by bending the leg that is forward at the knee joint. If you find it simple, draw back the knee of the bent leg as far as possible. The other leg should remain straight.

Pain can be expected at the back of the forward leg if the muscles are short there, and also close to the hip of the leg which is bent.

Chest Pump

Purpose: To develop the extensors of the elbow and trunk and the flexors and extensors of the hip on one side while exercising the flexors and extensors of the moving leg (knee and hip).

Position: Front leaning rest position as in push-ups.

Exercise: Bring the right knee up to the chest quickly and return without pause. Do not allow the right toe to touch the floor again after the exercise is started. Continue the movement, bringing the knee to the chest in a pumping action. Repeat on the opposite side. The exercise is done in two counts, or one count if done rapidly.

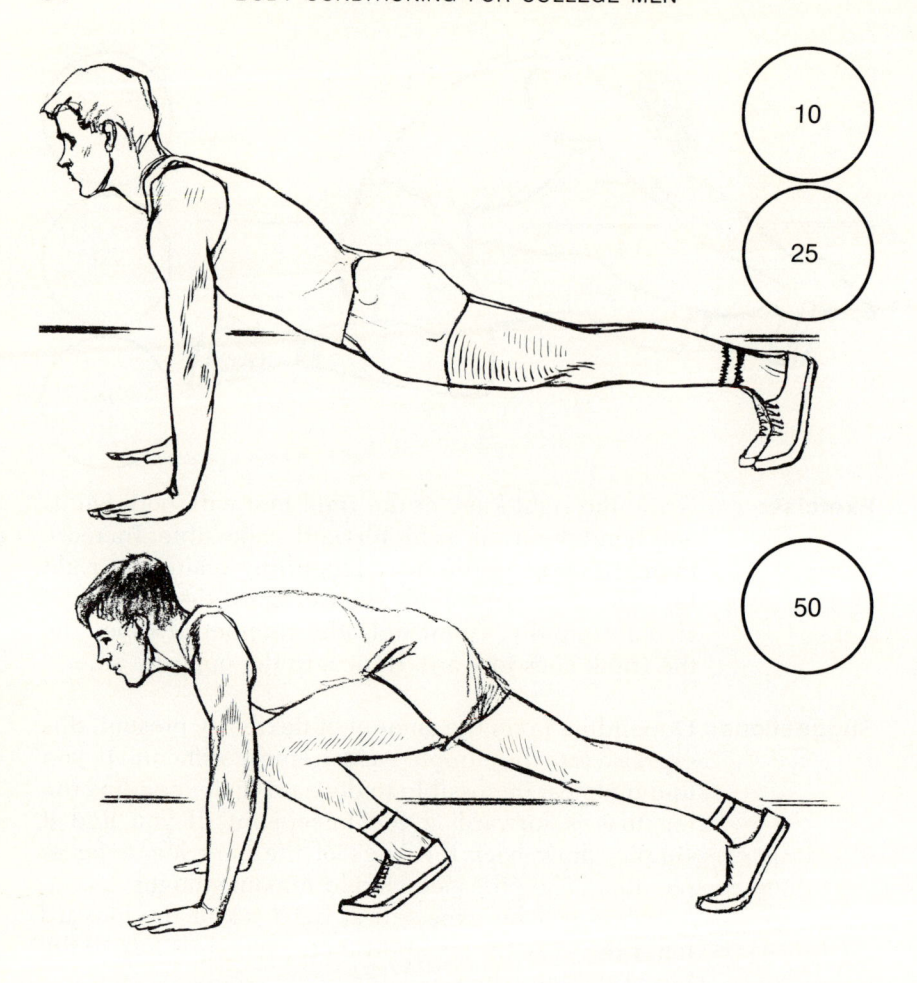

Suggestions: This is a simple movement which should be done with the hips kept in line with the shoulders and heels. Increased flexibility in the ankle joint may be aided by resting the stationary foot on the instep rather than on the toe.

The Frustrator

Purpose: To develop the flexor muscles of the neck and the hips and the extensors of the knees. The pectoral muscles

③ ⑤ ⑩

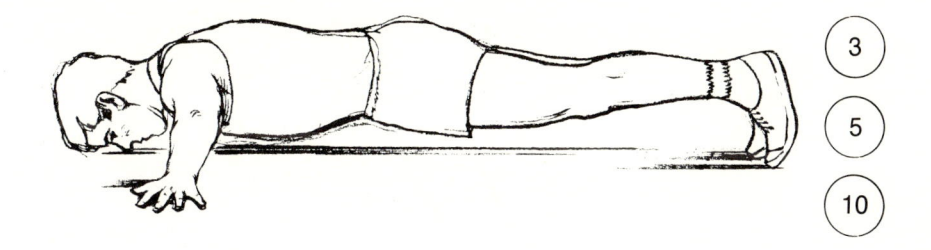

in the chest and the flexors of the elbow joint are also exercised.

Position: Lie face down with arms to side, horizontally, palms down. Feet should be kept apart.

Exercise: Press hands, toes and forehead against floor; tense entire body and try to raise it off the floor with the weight distributed on the hands, toes and forehead. The exercise can be done in four counts, up on one and two and down on three and four.

Suggestions: This is probably the most difficult exercise in any ordinary program of free exercise. For those who cannot get their hips off the floor, it will be of help to bring the hands in close to the chest. Those who cannot complete the movement can use it as an isometric exercise.

Bicycling

Purpose: To exercise the extensors of the hip and knee.

Position: Lie on back and extend legs overhead, resting only on the back of the head, neck, shoulders and elbows. With the elbows on the floor the hands can brace the hips.

Exercise: Alternate leg movement as though riding a bicycle. The movement can be as fast or slow as desired, but increased action will provide the most benefit.

Suggestions: Begin with slow movement and gradually increase the speed until the maximum is reached. Decrease the speed gradually and then increase it again. Alternate from slow to fast to slow several times.

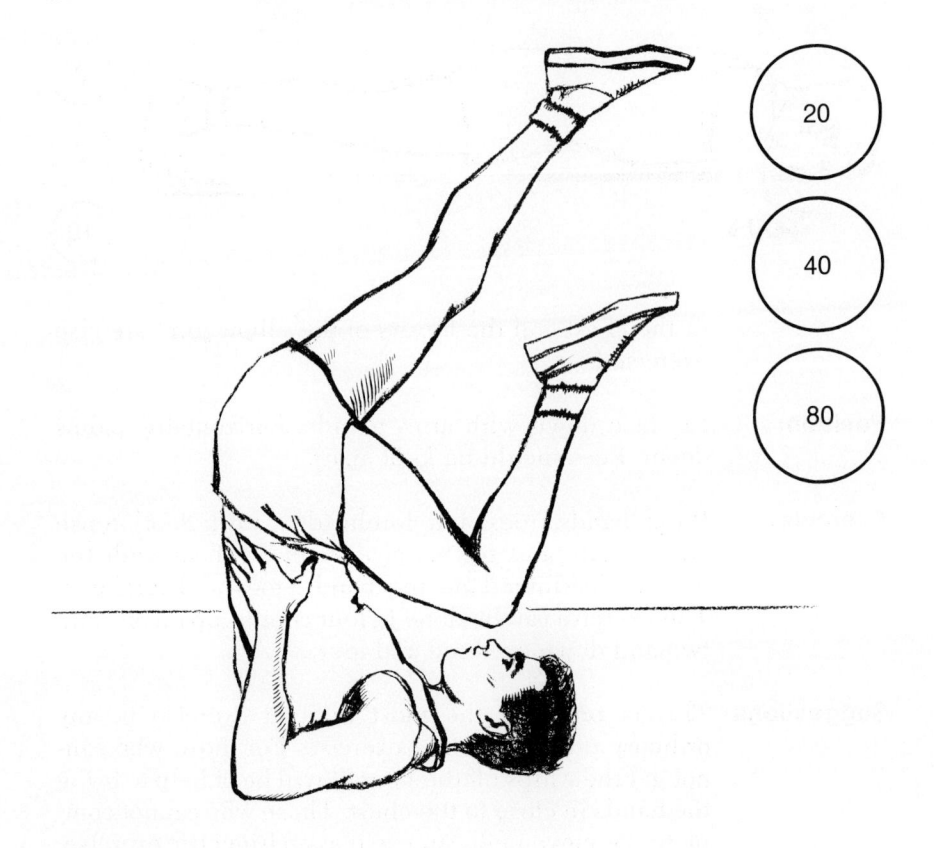

Duck-up

Purpose: To stretch the knee flexor muscles as well as to increase the flexibility of the lower back by stretching the latissimus dorsi (extensor) muscle.

Position: Squat, keeping the hands flat on the floor about six inches in front of the feet.

Exercise: Try to keep the hands flat on the floor and straighten the legs. Strain should be felt in the hamstring muscles in the backs of the legs.

Suggestions: If the strain is too great and the legs cannot be straightened completely, try the exercise with the fingertips touching the floor. Keep the fingertips on the floor and try to straighten the legs as much as possible.

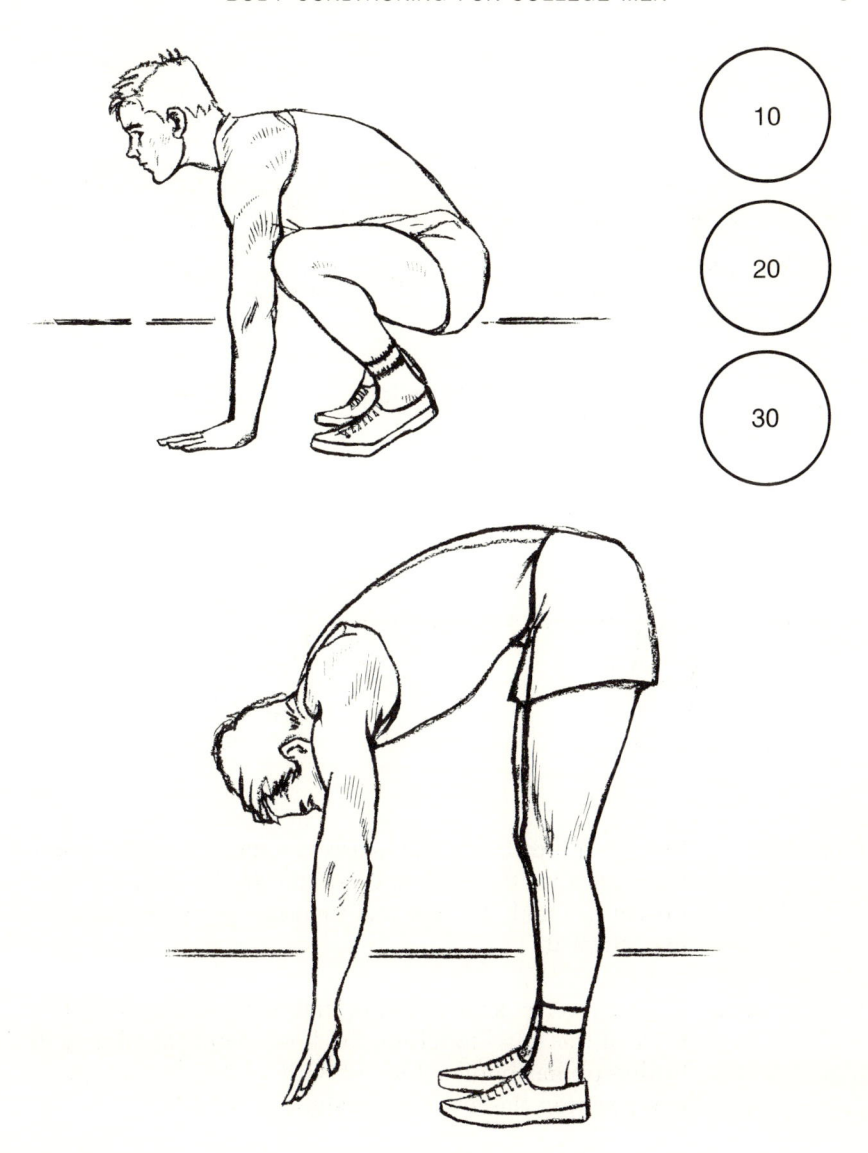

Bridge-up

Purpose: To increase flexibility in the back, hips and shoulders. The triceps muscle in the back of the arm is strengthened as a secondary effect.

Position: Lie on the back with the knees bent and the hands on the floor behind the shoulders.

38   BODY CONDITIONING FOR COLLEGE MEN

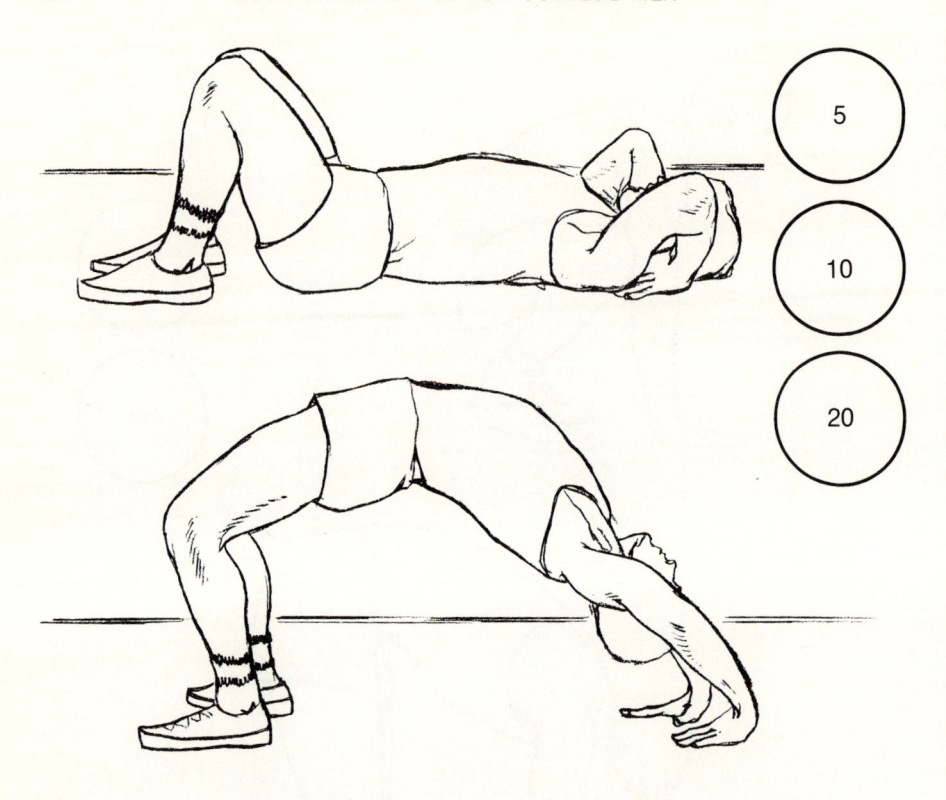

⬤ 5

⬤ 10

⬤ 20

Exercise: Bridge up until only the hands and feet are on the floor. Push up until the arms are straight on the count of one. Lower the body by bending the elbows on the count of two. Repeat.

Suggestions: If the exercise is too difficult, practice bridging with the back of the head touching the floor. After the ability to bridge up has been achieved with moderate skill, practice pushing the arms up straight.

Bounce

Purpose: To exercise the muscles that extend the hip joint (gluteus maximus and semitendinosus) and to stretch the pectoral muscles of the chest and the quadriceps muscles of the thigh.

Position: Back leaning rest position with the feet apart.

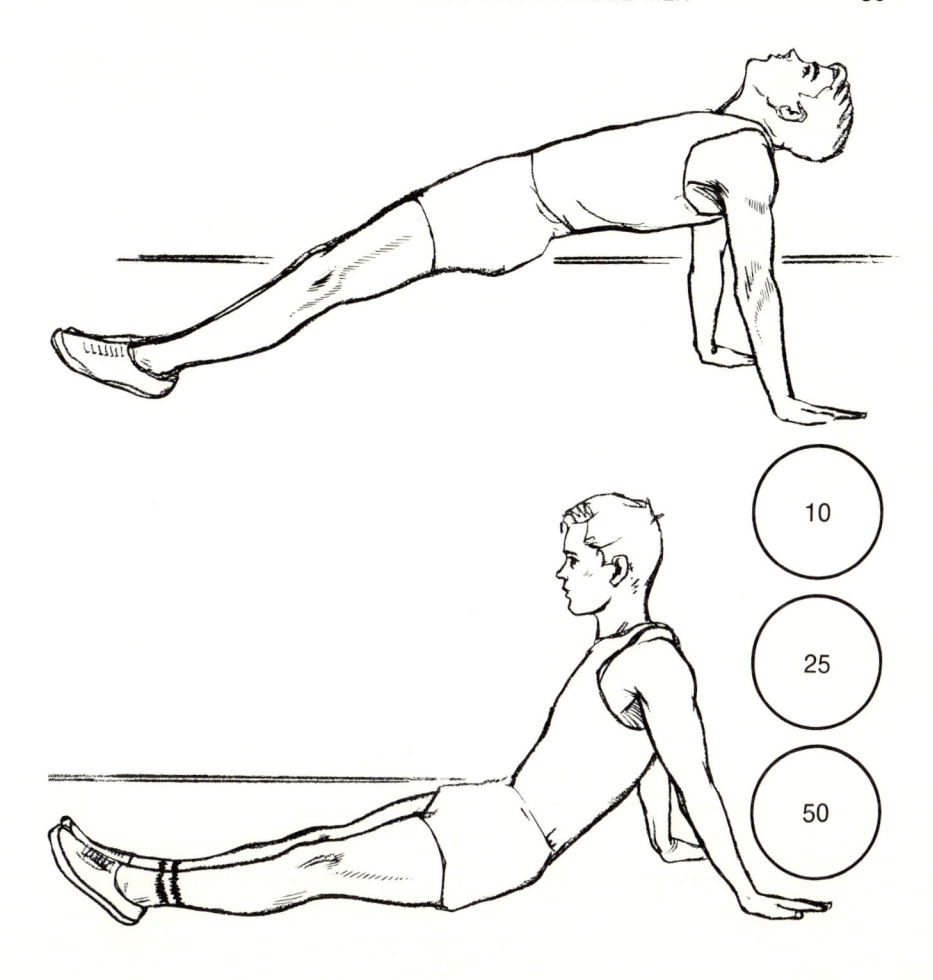

Exercise: Lower the hips almost to a sitting position and then raise them rapidly.

Suggestions: More action can be obtained by throwing the hips up with a vigorous movement until the heels are forced off the floor.

The Grinder

Purpose: To increase flexibility in the lower back and hips by stretching the erector spinae muscles and to strengthen the abdominal (rectus abdominis) and lateral trunk (internal and external oblique) muscles.

	5
	10
	20

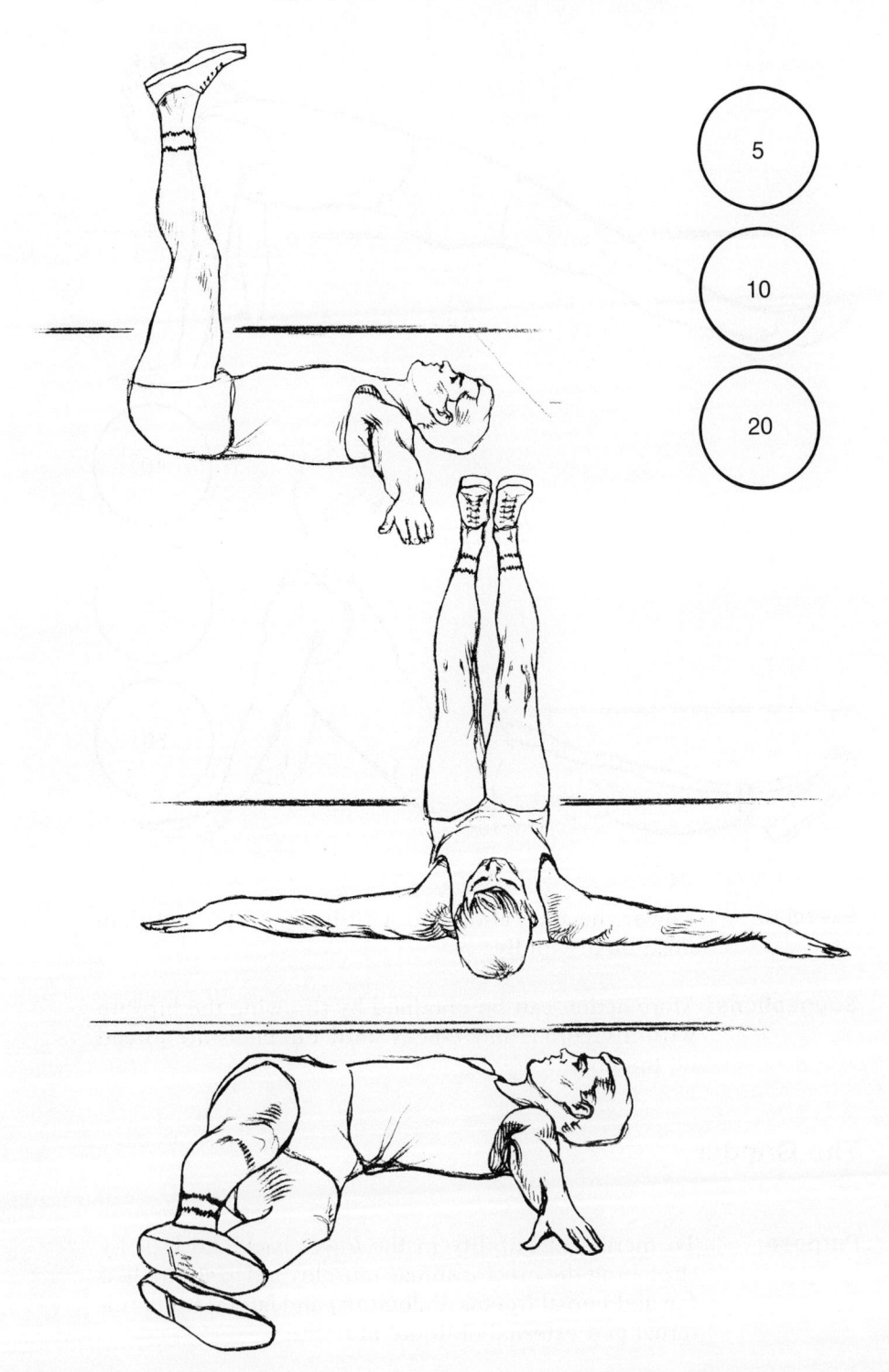

Position: Lie on the back with arms at the side in horizontal position and palms down. Lift the legs straight up in the vertical position. The back and hips should be flat on the floor.

Exercise: Lower both feet, keeping the ankles touching at all times, down to the left side until the outer border of left foot touches the floor. Press down with the left hand on the floor and raise both feet together to the vertical position again. Alternate on the other side. The shoulders should be kept flat at all times with the shoulder blades drawn back. Use four or eight counts for this exercise.

Suggestions: Body build may have some effect on the ease with which this exercise is done. Persons with short legs should have little difficulty, while those with long legs may find it hard to do properly. For the latter, the knees can be bent to decrease the gravity pull.

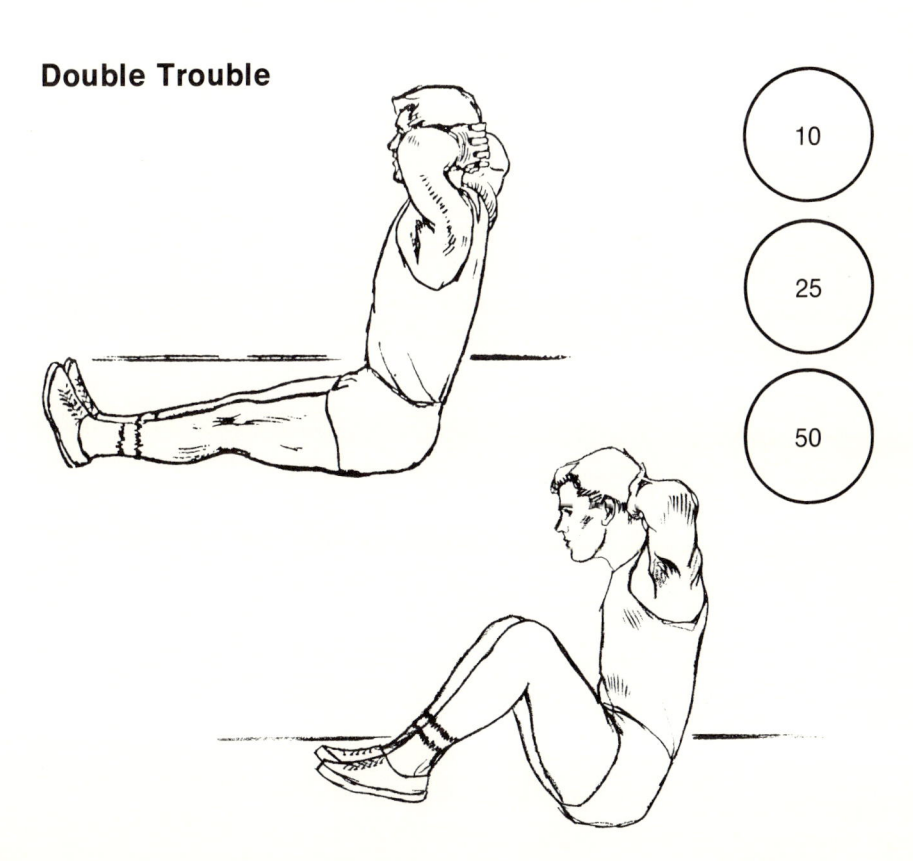

Double Trouble

10

25

50

Purpose: To exercise the hip and trunk flexor muscles and to stretch the chest (pectoralis) muscles. The extensors of the knee are also exercised. Maintenance of balance through muscular action is also accomplished.

Position: Sit with hands clasped behind head and elbows well back. Legs are extended straight forward.

Exercise: Raise both knees to the chest and return, using a count of two.

Suggestions: This exercise will be more difficult if the feet are not allowed to touch the floor from start to finish. This requires considerable balancing ability and keeps more muscle groups in constant action. Less difficulty will be encountered if the toes are allowed to drag on the floor.

UNIT III

NEW TRENDS IN EXERCISE
Isotonic Exercise
Isometric Exercise
THE BIG TEN: ISOMETRICS
A BUSY MAN'S SPECIAL
WEIGHT TRAINING
FLEXIBILITY EXERCISE
PULLEY WEIGHT EXERCISE

NEW TRENDS IN EXERCISE

Isometric and isotonic are terms applied to methods of exercising muscle groups. In the isometric method the muscles exert force by pushing or pulling against an immovable object. Isotonic exercise is characterized by the exertion of force on a movable object, such as the weights used in weight training, or on other parts of the body, as occurs in sit-ups. Both methods increase muscular strength, and both have been shown to bring about significant gains in strength sooner than other methods.

Isotonic Exercise

Isotonic exercises involve muscular contraction and movement is produced. The greatest advantage of isotonic over isometric exercise is that the former develops the muscles over a range of motion while the latter has a tendency to increase the strength of the muscle greatly only at the angle at which it was exercised. There seems to be a psychological advantage to the isotonic method, for many people find it less boring than static exercise. Like the isometric exercises, the isotonic exercises need to be supplemented with other activities to provide for the development of all the components of physical fitness.

Isometric Exercise

Isometric exercises are excellent for developing power and strength. Participants in football, track, wrestling and gymnastics (sports in which power and strength are essential for effective performance) have used isometric exercises to excellent advantage. The isometrics are also beneficial in redeveloping power and strength of muscles that have been debilitated by injury or illness. They have proved particularly useful to people with physical handicaps because they do not involve the complex and highly coordinated movements of many other kinds of exercises which such people are unable or too embarrassed to perform. Because these exercises require no equipment, little space and relatively little time, they are an excellent substitute for the regular exerciser who must forego his daily routine because of travel or pressure of work.

There is little shortening or contraction of the muscles and no appreciable movement in the performance of isometric exercise. Consequently, no significant development of coordination, flexibility and endurance occurs. Because of these limitations, isometric exercise should not be the only form; other forms that necessitate vigorous movements are needed to ensure a total workout for the body.

There are two separate sets of isometric exercises on the following pages, called the Big Ten and A Busy Man's Special. Experiment with both sets and choose those exercises that best fit your particular needs. In doing the exercises, hold each position for six seconds, and follow it with six seconds of rest. Repeat each exercise five or six times. Try to finish each session by jogging in place to stimulate circulation.

THE BIG TEN: ISOMETRICS

The Arm Lift

Purpose: To exercise the flexor muscles of the elbow and wrist joints and, of secondary importance, the extensors of the back and legs and the forward section of the deltoid, located in the shoulder area.

Position: Stand with feet slightly apart and grasp the edge of a desk or countertop which is immovable. Brace yourself firmly, keeping back and legs in a fixed position.

Exercise: Attempt to lift the object by trying to flex the elbow joint.

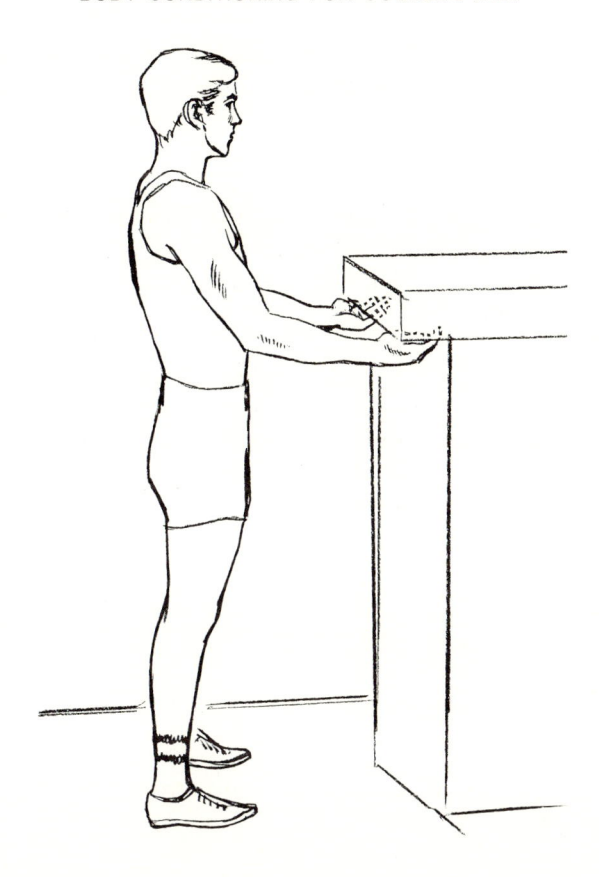

Suggestions: Since the main effort here is to exercise the arms, a good fixed position of the trunk and legs is important. The natural tendency is to involve all the lifting muscles, including those of the legs and back. Even though it is impossible to isolate groups of muscles entirely when exercising, it is important in this case to forego raising the heels from the floor or extending the hips.

The Leg Lift

Purpose: To exercise the extensor muscles of the hip and knee joint and, secondarily, of the back, which act in a supporting role.

Position: Stand with back straight and arms hanging down; place hands under any immovable object. The knees must be bent and the object upon which force is to be exerted must be lower than the natural level of the hands.

Exercise: Keeping the back and arms straight, place the hands under the object to be lifted. When the lifting position has been assumed and the feet are firmly positioned for maximum effort, an attempt is made to straighten the knees. The trunk and the arms are held as straight as possible.

Suggestions: First be sure that the object upon which the force is to be expended is safely anchored. When the lift is to be attempted and the feet are firmly set, experiment to be sure that no slipping will occur. Make the lift in as straight an up and down position as possible.

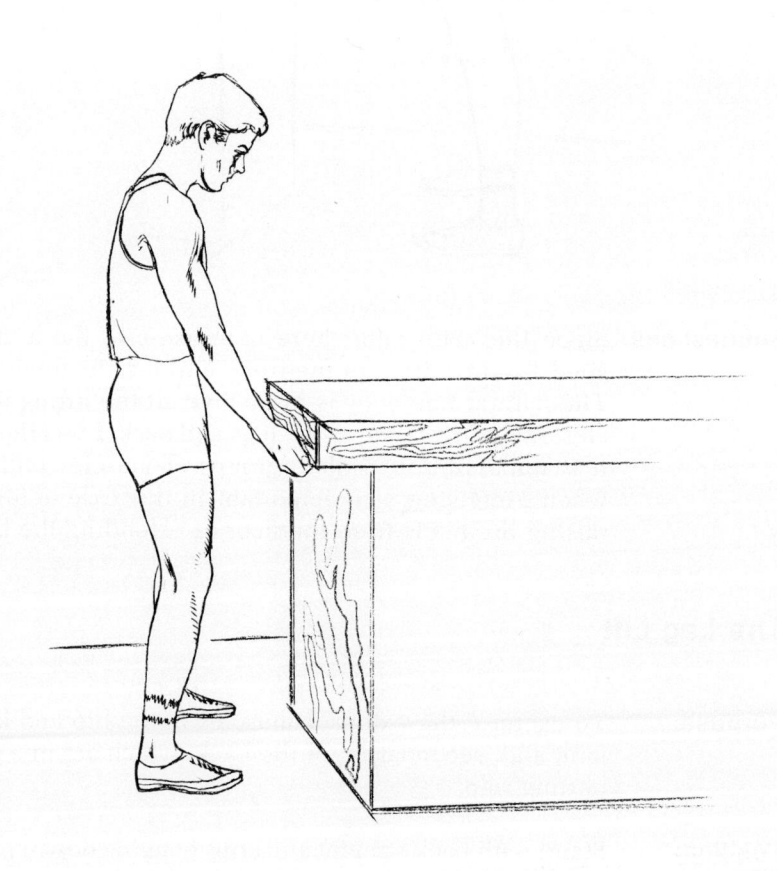

Arm Depression

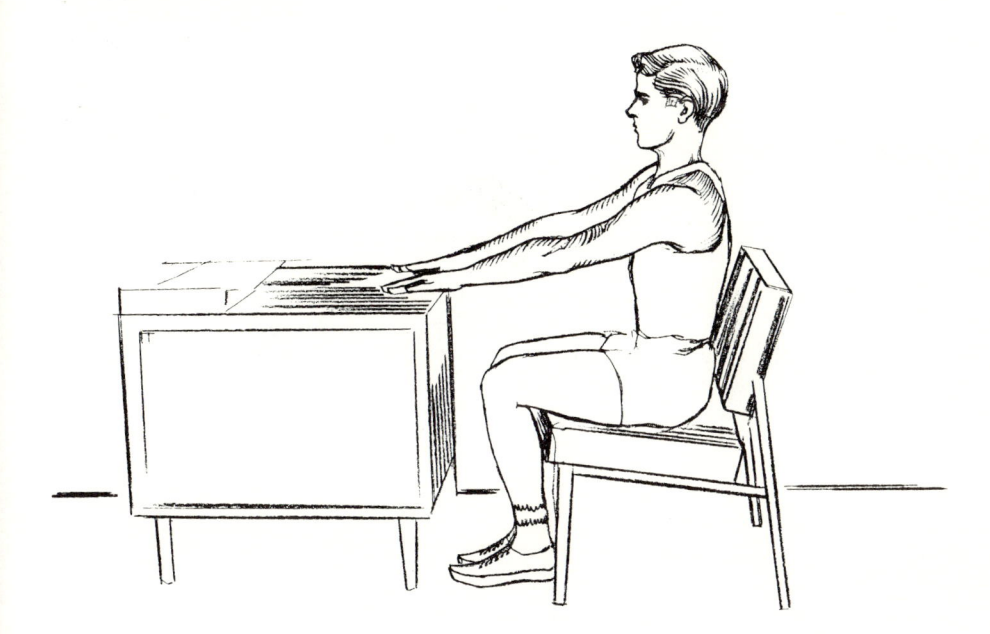

Purpose: To develop those muscles which depress the arms and, secondarily, the extensors of the elbow and the flexors of the wrist and fingers.

Position: Sit or stand with arms extended and with the palms of the hands on the top of a table, desk, dresser or file cabinet.

Exercise: Keeping the elbow and wrist joints in full extension, press downward with the hands. The trunk is held upright.

Suggestions: The natural tendency here is to rise from the chair when the downward pressure of the arms is first begun. To eliminate this reaction, make a direct effort to bend the trunk forward for the first few attempts. Once you get the "feel" of the exercise, you are better able to hold the trunk in the desired position and to apply the most force.

Elbow Extension

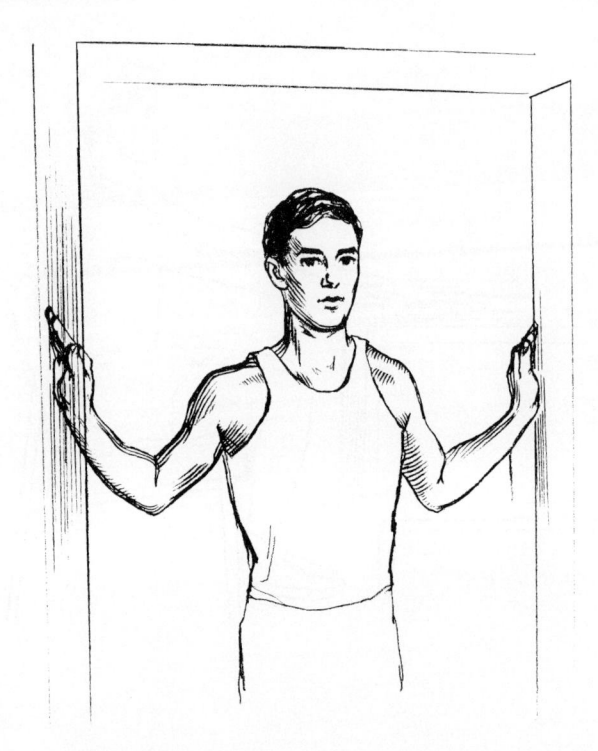

Purpose: To develop the triceps, the only major muscle used in extending the elbow joint. One small muscle, the anconeus, assists mildly in this action. In the position suggested, the deltoid is also exercised.

Position: Stand in the center of the doorway and place the palms of both hands against the two sides of the door frame at shoulder level.

Exercise: Push against the sides of the frame with equal pressure from each arm. Try to extend the arms at the elbow joints.

Suggestions: A comfortable stance must be taken to achieve the maximum benefit from this exercise. A wide door frame is more suitable than a narrow one as a cramped position will not allow for proper leverage. If only a narrow space is available, better leverage can be had by placing the back against one side of the frame and pushing with both hands against the other.

Shoulders (Arm Abduction)

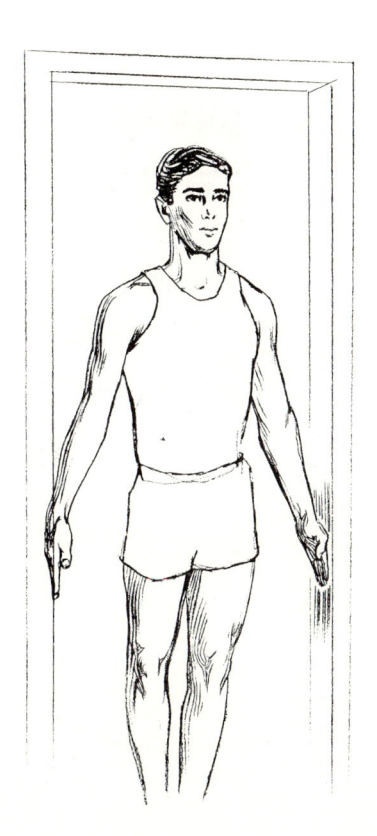

Purpose: To develop the muscles involved in elevation of the upper arm, with the deltoid as the prime mover. Extensors of the elbow and wrist joints provide secondary action.

Position: Stand in the center of doorway; place backs of hands against door frame at hip level. Keep arms straight and fix the wrists.

Exercise: Try to raise arms sideward and upward.

Suggestions: A narrow door frame is to be preferred for this exercise. If there is no suitable frame available, you may exercise one arm at a time by standing close to a wall with the legs spread and the body leaning toward the wall.

Upper Back and Shoulders

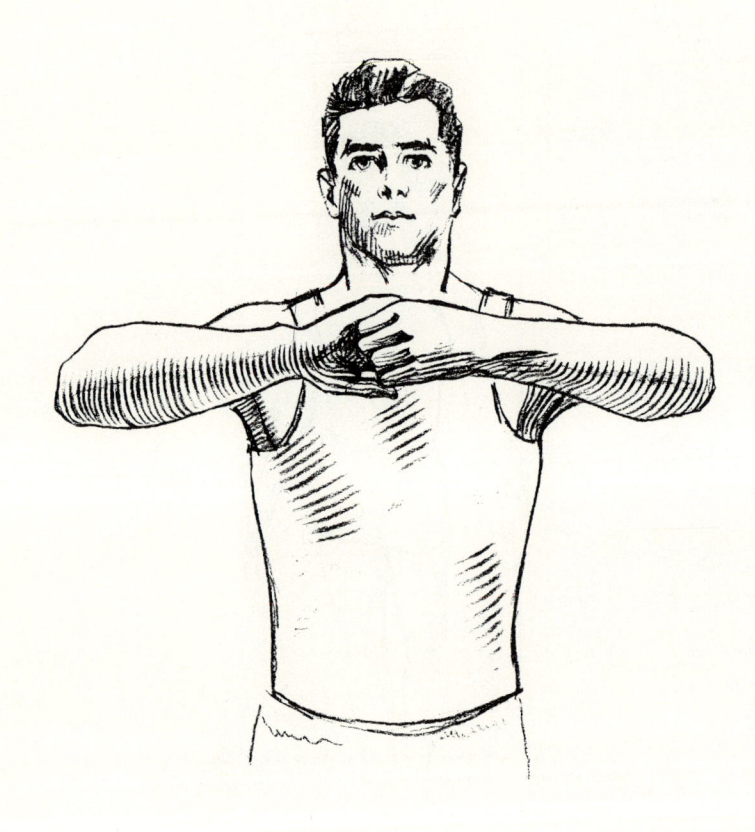

Purpose: To develop the adductors of the shoulders. Secondary action involves the elbow extensors and the flexors of the fingers.

Position: Stand or sit with hands at chest level and elbows raised to same level as hands. Reverse one hand and lock fingertips.

Exercise: Try to pull elbows backward, keeping fingers locked.

Suggestions: If the fingers are not strong enough to hold, the same position can be attained by grasping each wrist. The best action is achieved by holding the elbows up high or as near the level of the shoulders as possible.

Chest

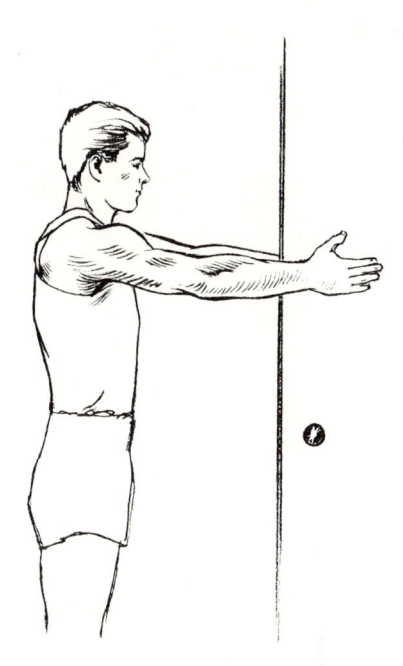

Purpose: To develop the muscles of the chest with the pectoralis major as the prime mover. Secondarily, the flexors of the elbows and the wrists are exercised.

Position: Stand in front of an object on which force can be exerted on two sides, raise arms forward and up to chest level, elbows extended. Place palms of hands on each side.

Exercise: Try to bring the hands together, squeezing the object between the hands.

Suggestions: The best action is obtained if only the hands are in contact with the object. The knees, elbows and hips should remain straight so that most of the pull is on the chest muscles.

Arms (Depression Sideward Plane)

Purpose: To develop those muscles involved in arm depression, such as the latissimus dorsi and the downward rotators of the scapula. Secondary action involves extensors of the elbow and the flexors of the fingers.

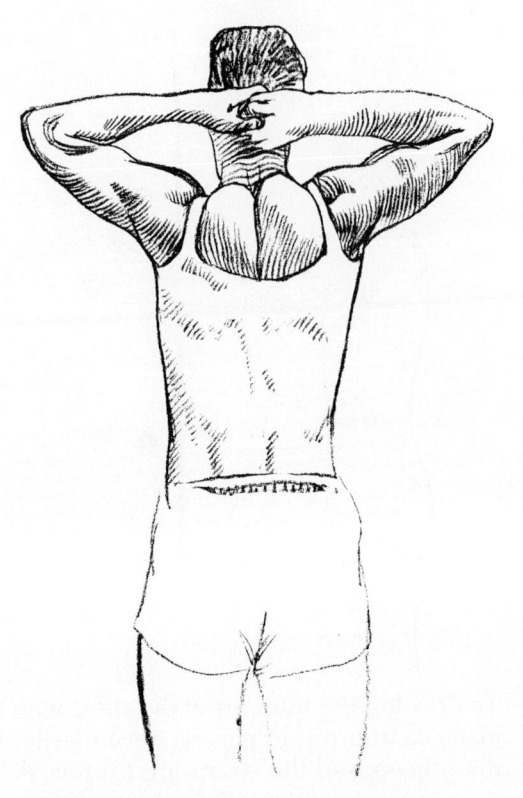

Position: Stand or sit, and raise both hands to front or back of head. Reverse one hand and lock fingertips together. Keep elbows sideward at the same level as the hands.

Exercise: Try to bring the elbows sideward and down while keeping the fingers locked.

Suggestions: A door frame may be substituted for the finger grasp. If a sitting position is assumed, the arms can be held over the head with the palms against each side of the frame. In this instance, greater stress is placed on the elbow extensors than on the muscles that depress the arm.

Hips (Sideward Movement of Legs)

Purpose: To develop those muscles which are used in leg abduction.

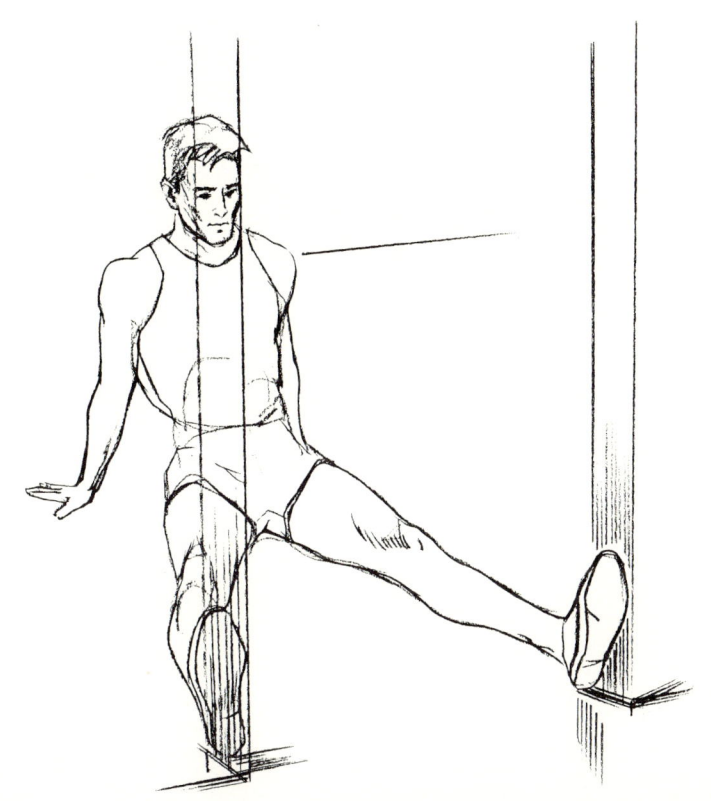

Position: Sit at a desk with the outer border of the knees against the desk frame, or in a narrow doorway with the outer border of the legs or ankles against the door frame. Try to obtain a space in which the legs will not be too far apart.

Exercise: Press outward against the desk or door frame with knees or ankles.

Suggestions: Two other ways to perform this exercise are: (1) to sit by a wall and press one leg at a time against the wall and (2) to lie on one side and raise the top leg upward against an immovable object.

Hips (Inward Movement of Legs)

Purpose: To develop those leg muscles which adduct (bring the legs together). This is a particularly good exercise for those who ski, skate or wrestle.

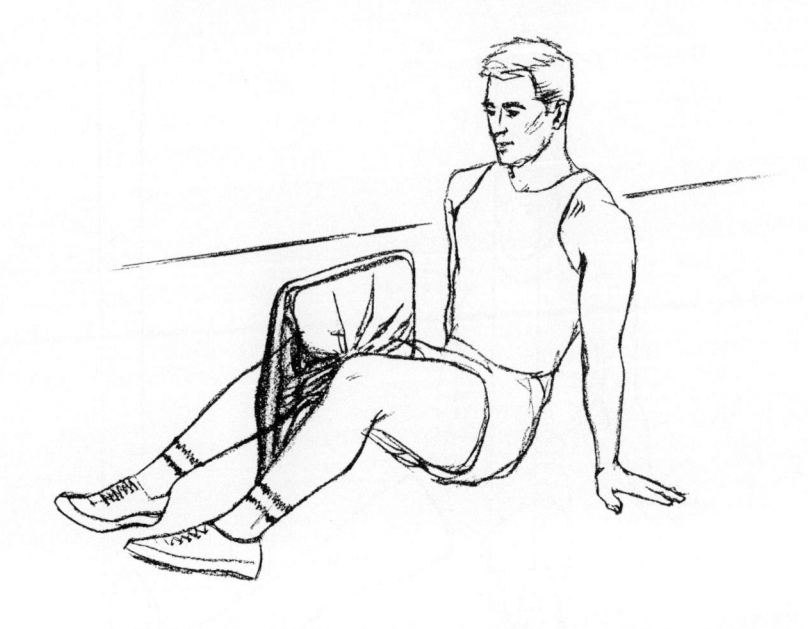

Position: Sit or lie with the inner border of the knees or ankles against a pillow, cushion, file cabinet or similar object.

Exercise: Squeeze legs together.

Suggestions: A sitting position with the hands placed on the floor in back of the hips seems to be the most effective position for this exercise. Pillows or cushions between the knees afford the greatest comfort. The same muscles can be exercised by strapping the ankles to immovable objects that hold the feet about 24 inches apart and then squeezing the legs together.

A BUSY MAN'S SPECIAL

The following exercises form a pattern which helps to strengthen groups of muscles in the neck, shoulders, chest, abdomen and legs. They are supplementary exercises and should not be used in place of the Daily Dozen or the Double Dozen exercises given earlier, but they may be used if time or convenience will not permit a standard workout. All the following can be done in a sitting position. Push or pull in one direction is cancelled by exerting equal pressure in the opposite direction.

Head Press Sideward

Purpose: To develop the muscles on the side of the neck (sternocleidomastoid and scalenus) and the upper part of the back (trapezius). The deltoids (elevators of the arm) and biceps (flexors of the elbow) are also exercised.

Position: Sit or stand.

Exercise: Press palm of hand against side of head and at the same time resist by pushing the head sideways against the hand. Repeat on the opposite side. Hold pressure for a count of six. Relax for a count of six.

Suggestions: Considerable care should be taken when exercising the neck region. Apply pressure lightly for the first few times until a feel for the correct amount of force is attained.

Head Press Forward

Purpose: To develop the sternocleidomastoid muscles, which draw the head forward. This also develops the biceps and deltoids of the shoulders and arms.

Position: Sit or stand.

Exercise: Press both hands against the forehead and counter-press by pushing the head forward and down.

Suggestions: Try holding the arms rigid and pressing the forehead into the hands. As you progress, exert equal forces both ways.

Head Press Backward

Purpose: To strengthen the back of the neck (trapezius and assisting muscles), the rhomboids (which elevate the scapula) and the pectorals (chest muscles).

Position: Sit or stand.

Exercise: Press both hands to the back of the head. Counter the pressure of the hands by forcing the head back with equal pressure.

Suggestions: Slightly more pressure can be exerted in back than in front, as the muscles in the back of the neck are stronger. Again, however, proceed with caution.

Leg Extension Arm Pull

Purpose: To increase the strength of the leg extensors, the elbow flexors and the abdominal muscles (rectus abdominis).

Position: Sit with knees bent.

Exercise: Grasp both ankles and pull back, bringing the heels toward the buttocks. Counter the pull of the arms by extending both legs with equal force.

Suggestions: Vary the position of the legs so that action can be developed with the knees at more than one angle of flexion or extension.

Leg Adduction

Purpose: To develop the leg adductors.

Position: Sit with knees bent and cross the arms. The hands are pressed against the inner side of each knee, the right hand against the left knee and vice versa.

Exercise: Try to bring both knees together, while resisting with hand pressure.

Suggestions: Keep pressure constant. A sandbag or similar aid may be used in place of hand pressure.

Leg Abduction

Purpose: To strengthen the leg abductors.

Position: Sit with knees bent and with the hands against the outsides of the knees.

Exercise: Spread knees apart. Push in with the hands while resisting with the knees.

Suggestions: If the trunk is lowered to a position where the chest is close to the thighs, greater leverage can be exerted against the legs. This may not be wise at the beginning, but it will be more effective when the legs begin to strengthen.

Arm Depression

Purpose: To develop the flexors of the fingers, the extensors of the wrists and the lower rhomboids and latissimus dorsi muscles, which help to depress the arm.

Position: Stand, sit or lie supine. The arms are extended overhead with fingers clasped together.

Exercise: Without releasing the fingers, try to bring the arms sideward and downward.

Suggestions: If one arm is rotated outward with the palm of the hand facing up and the fingers curled, a good grip can be secured with the fingers of the other hand and they will be locked together tightly.

WEIGHT TRAINING

Weight training, or isotonic exercise with weights, is used in conditioning programs chiefly for the development of strength. It has been used very successfully in athletic training to develop the explosive strength so essential in sports participation. Programs of weight training have also been used effectively in the rehabilitation of injured muscles and to increase strength during the convalescent period after a long illness. For the person interested in improving his physical fitness, weight training provides a means of developing strength.

For the performance of weight training exercises, bars, weights or weighted objects are necessary. The need for special equipment may be considered an inconvenience by some, but others find its use more interesting and stimulating than performing exercise without equipment.

How to begin

Until you have become experienced enough with the exercises to create your own routine, begin with the first exercise (page 58) and do each exercise in the order in which it is presented.

For each exercise, select a weight you think you can lift about ten times in succession without fatigue. Attempt the exercise as described, paying special attention to any suggestions that are made regarding safety in making the lift. If you are able to lift the weight ten times without tiring, stop and add more weight so that when you start again you are able to do approximately ten repetitions before fatigue sets in. If, on the other hand, you have started the exercise with a weight so heavy that you cannot lift it ten times in succession without tiring, stop at the point of fatigue and for the next workout make the weight light enough so that you are able to do ten repetitions.

Having determined the suitable weight, use it in subsequent workouts until you can perform the exercises without strain; now you are ready to increase the amount of weight. You should attempt eight to ten repetitions of an exercise, resting for a few minutes between each series of repetitions. When you are able, you should repeat the entire ten exercises, doing ten repetitions of each.

When doing any of the weight training exercises, keep your body in good position, that is, a straight alignment of the body—head erect, chin up, chest high, abdomen sucked in, shoulders depressed, back straight, pelvis rotated (down in back, up in front) and legs parallel.

Precautions to observe in weightlifting are:
1. Never attempt an all-out lift without having first warmed up.
2. Use spotters when lifting heavy weights.
3. Always make certain that collars on weights are in position and are tight.
4. When lifting in a group, never lift over someone lying on the floor.
5. In moving heavy weights from one place to another or to and from the rack, lift from the crouch position (knees bent and back straight) to avoid straining the back.

Curls

Purpose: To strengthen the flexor muscles of the upper arm, an important group of muscles for lifting objects. These muscles are also among the prime movers in lifting one's own weight.

Position: Stand, holding weight against the thighs with hands palm up.

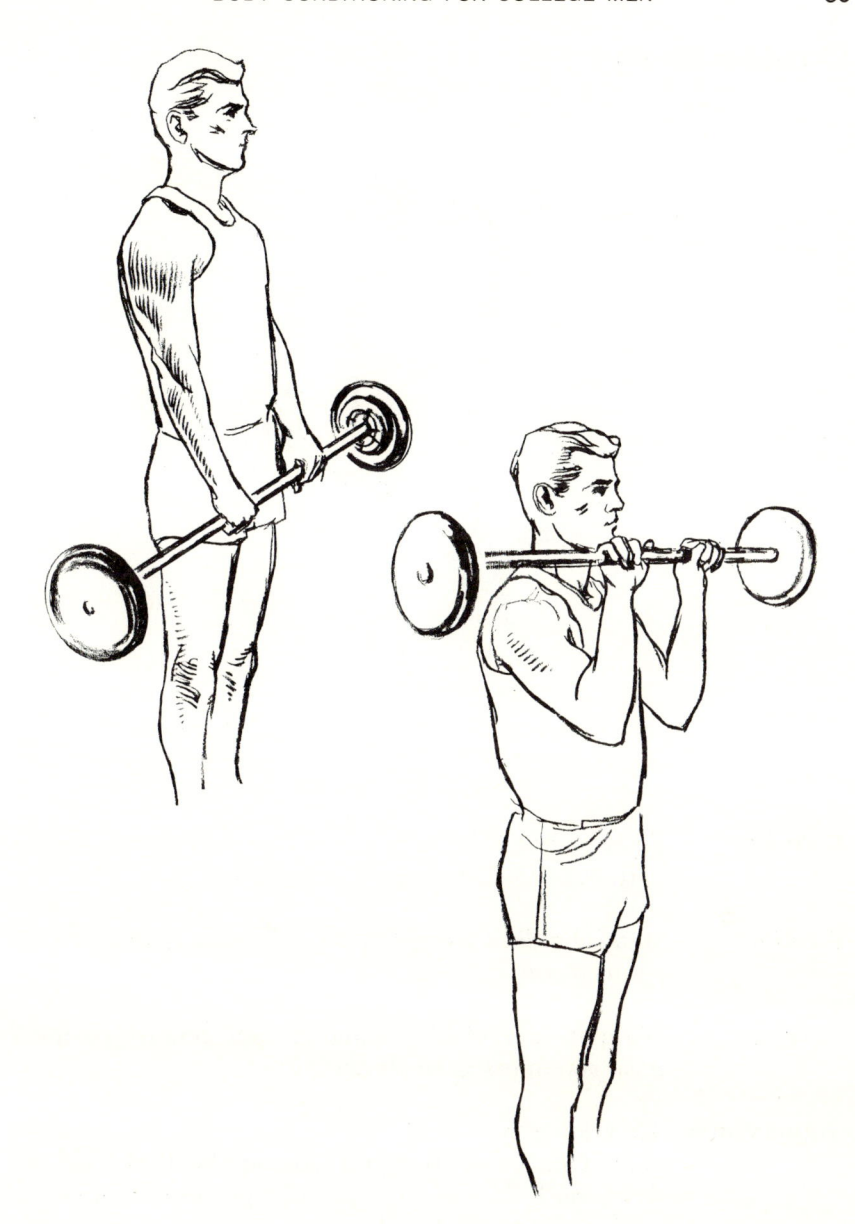

Exercise: Bend arms at elbow joints, raising weights to the chest-shoulder area. The trunk should be kept in an erect position during the exercise, and the elbows should be kept close to the ribs.

Suggestions: Chinning, bent arm hang and pulley weight curls may be substituted for this lift.

Shoulder Shrug

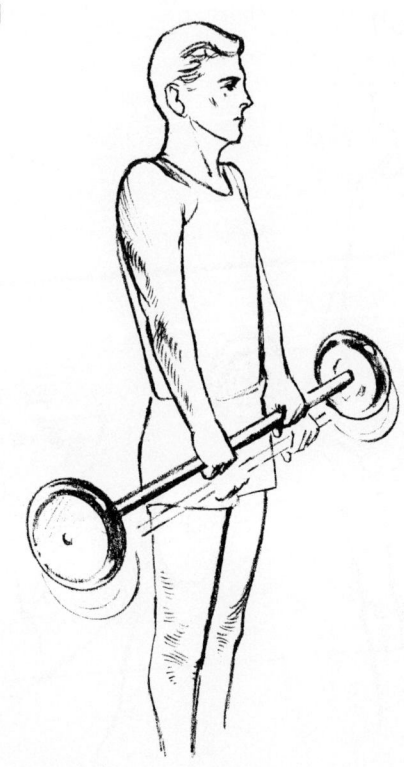

Purpose: To strengthen the upper back and shoulder area (deltoid, trapezius and levator scapularis).

Position: Stand, holding weight at arms' length against thighs, palms down.

Exercise: Without appreciably changing your general position, raise shoulders as in shrugging.

Suggestions: After doing the "shrug" a few times, rotate the shoulder joint. This will tend to pull the scapulae backward and downward. This is an excellent postural exercise as well as a strength builder.

Knee Bends

Purpose: To strengthen the extensors of the knee, important for lifting, walking upstairs and other common tasks. The exercise involves the muscles of the hip joint (gluteus maximus), the hamstrings, the knee joint (quadriceps) and the ankle joint (gastrocnemius, soleus).

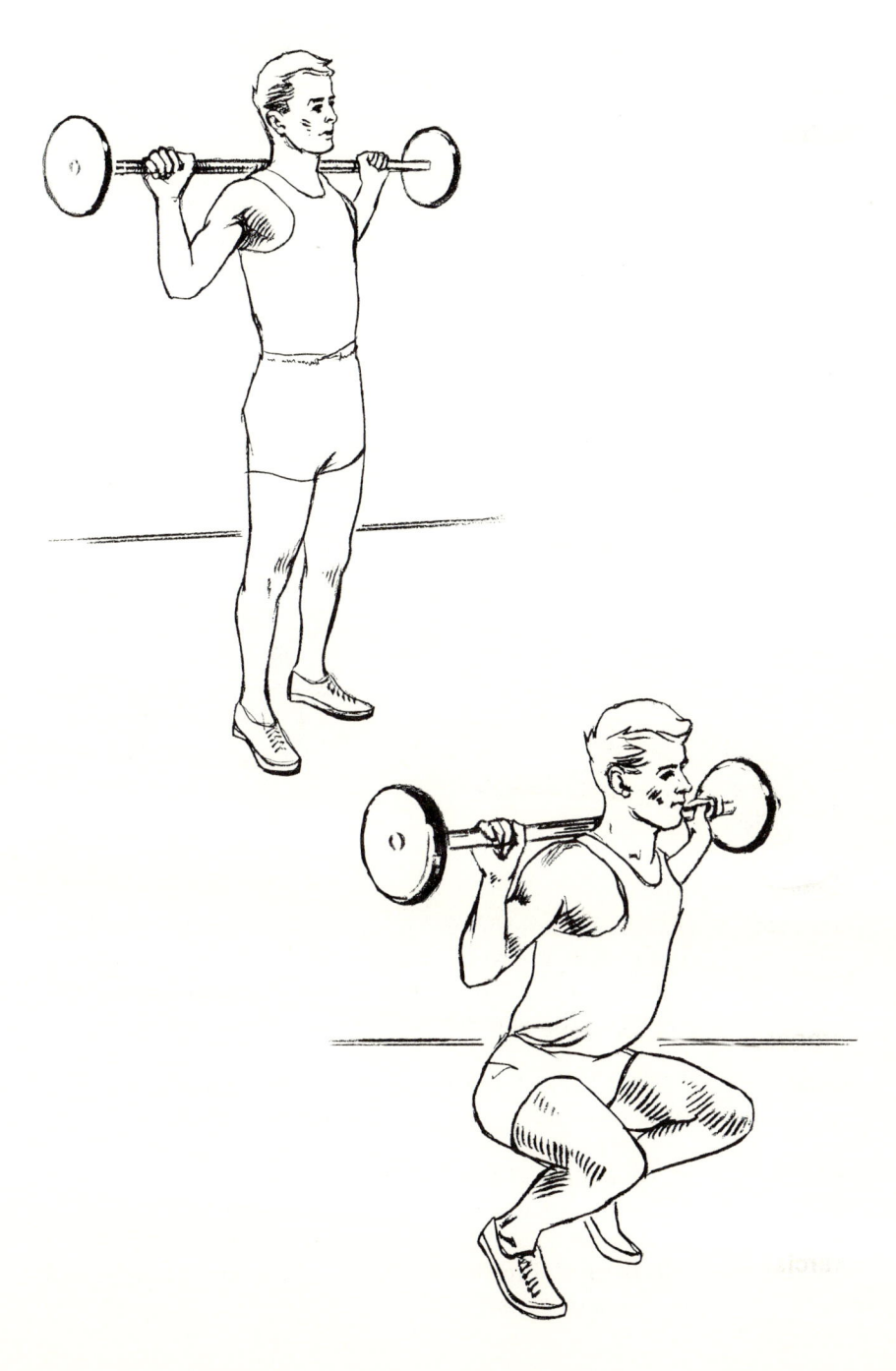

Position: Stand, holding weight across shoulders at back of neck.

Exercise: Rise on balls of feet; bend knees nearly to a half-squat.

Suggestions: The exercise can be done with someone of your general size on your back as in "pig-a-back." In order to bring the ankle joint into play, a board of about one or two inches in height may be put under the forward part of the feet. Raise the heel and return to position. This will strengthen the calf muscles. Anyone with knee difficulty should not bend more than a one-third squat, but instead may use a heavier weight.

Sit-ups

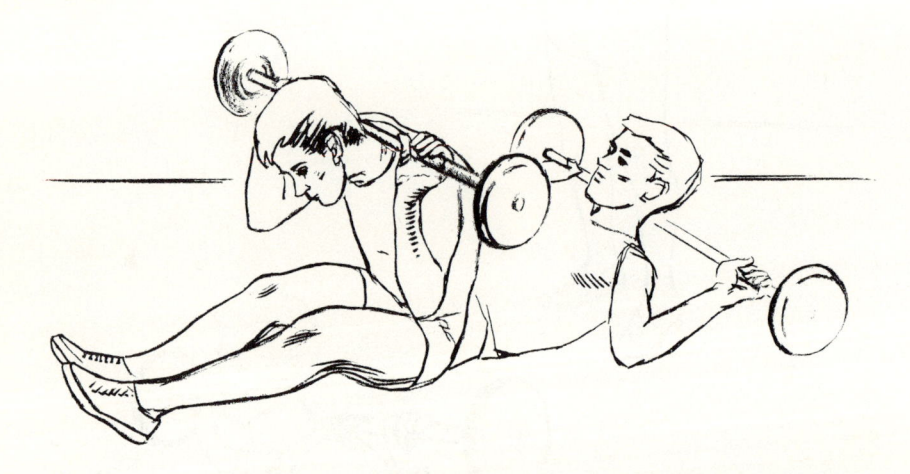

Purpose: To strengthen the abdominal muscles and hip flexors. If the legs are kept straight, the abdominals are only partially involved. If the knees are bent during the exercise, the abdominals do most of the work.

Position: Lie on back, holding weight across shoulders and in back of neck.

Exercise: Raise head and lift shoulders to bring upper body to a half sitting position. Keep legs straight.

Suggestions: Alternate doing this exercise with knees straight and with knees flexed.

Straight Arm Pullover with Bench Press

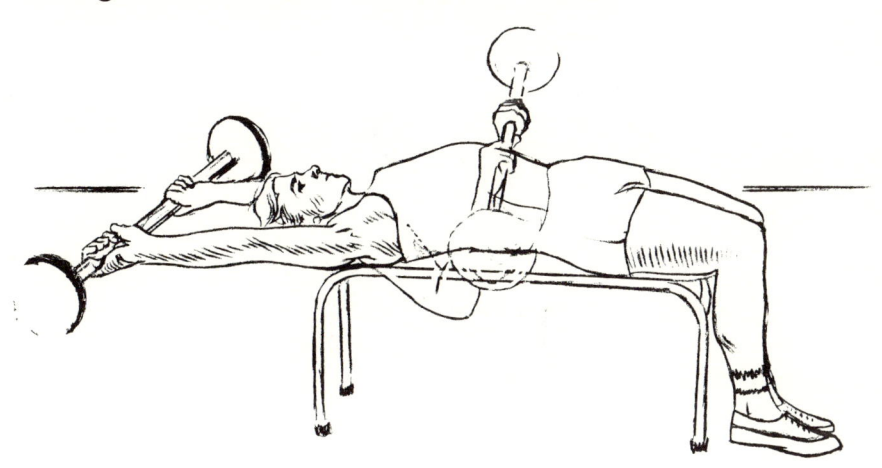

Purpose: To strengthen the shoulder and chest area, which includes the muscles affecting the shoulder joint (pectoralis major, latissimus dorsi), the shoulder girdle (serratus anterior, pectoralis minor) and the arms (triceps, anterior deltoid, coracobrachialis).

Position: Lie on back on bench with weight over the head at arms' length.

Exercise: Lift weight with straight arms to vertical position. Bend arms and bring weight to chest. Extend arms and return to position.

Suggestions: Start with light weight. Be careful not to go beyond the vertical position as you may lose control of the weight. If a second person is present, he can assist in relieving you of the weight when necessary and at the end of the exercise.

Trunk Bend

Purpose: To strengthen the extensor muscles affecting the lower back and hips (gluteus maximus, hamstrings and erector spinae groups).

Position: Stand with weight across shoulders behind neck.

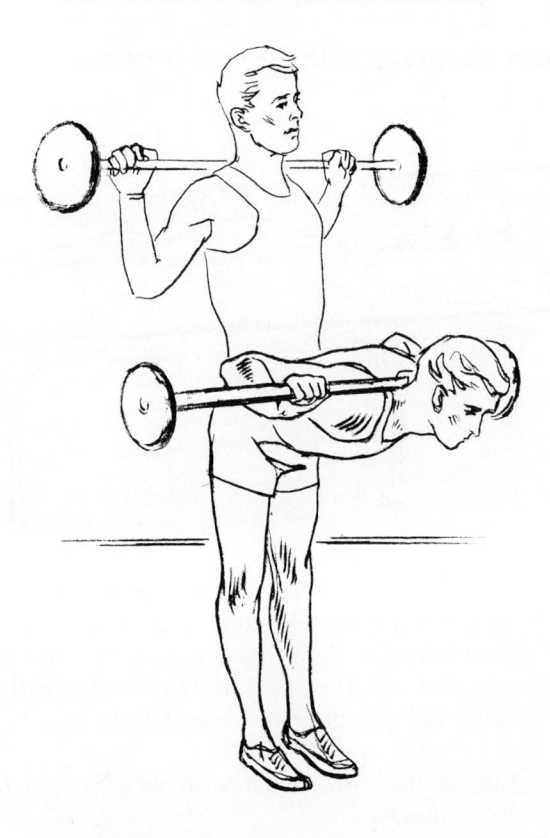

Exercise: Bend forward at the waist until the upper body is parallel to the floor. Return slowly to original position.

Suggestions: Do the exercise slowly. Allow the spine to straighten gradually from bottom to top by keeping the head and shoulders bent forward until the lower portion of the trunk is erect. This will strengthen the shoulder muscles that aid in maintaining good posture.

Lateral Raise

Purpose: To exercise the muscles affecting the shoulder joint (supraspinatus, deltoid, trapezius and serratus anterior).

Position: Stand with dumbbells or weights at sides.

Exercise: Raise weights (with straight arms) sideward and upward until arms are parallel with floor and shoulder high.

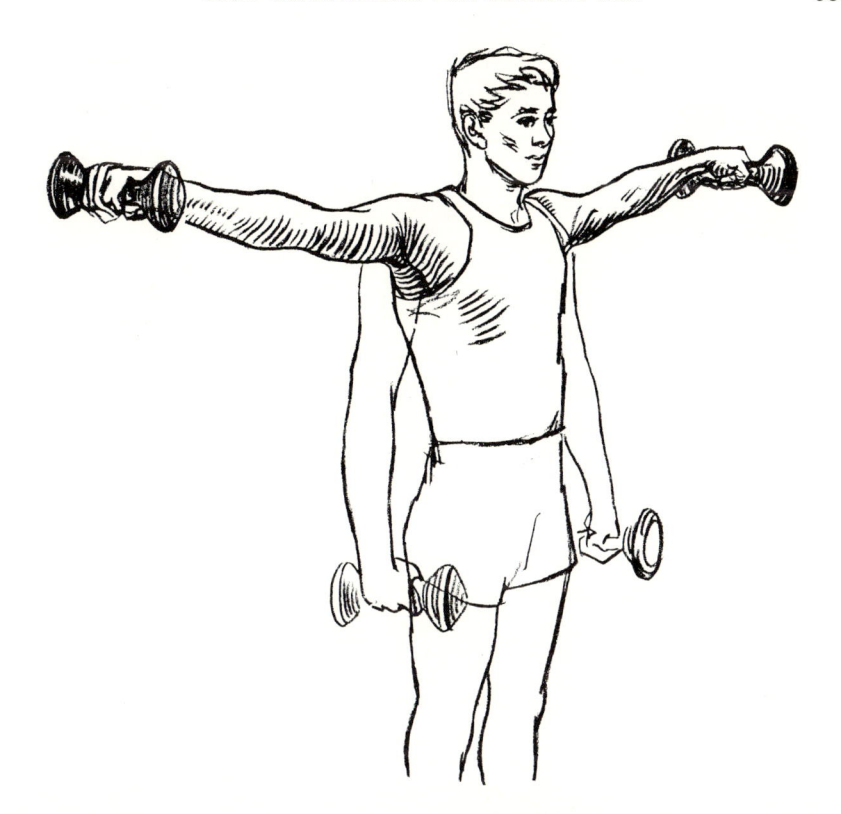

Suggestions: Keep body erect, chest high, abdomen high and pelvis rotated down in back and up in front. Keep palms of hands down.

Wings (Prone)

Purpose: To develop the upper back (a neglected area), the shoulder retractors (rhomboid and trapezius) and the posterior portions of the shoulder muscles (deltoids).

Position: Lie prone on a bench with arms down toward floor, holding weights.

Exercise: Raise arms sideward and upward until parallel to floor.

Suggestions: Be careful not to overload arms on this exercise. The back muscles are not always ready for hard work and back injury can result. On the other hand, strengthening the back muscles tends to eliminate back troubles.

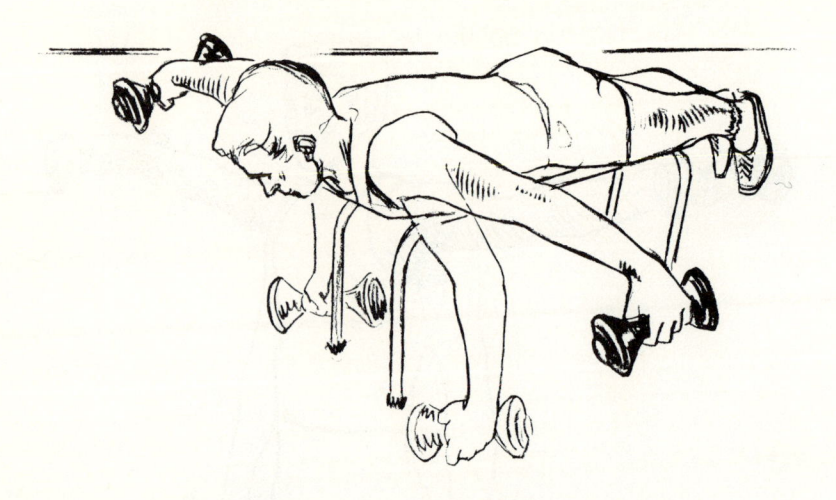

Wings (Supine)

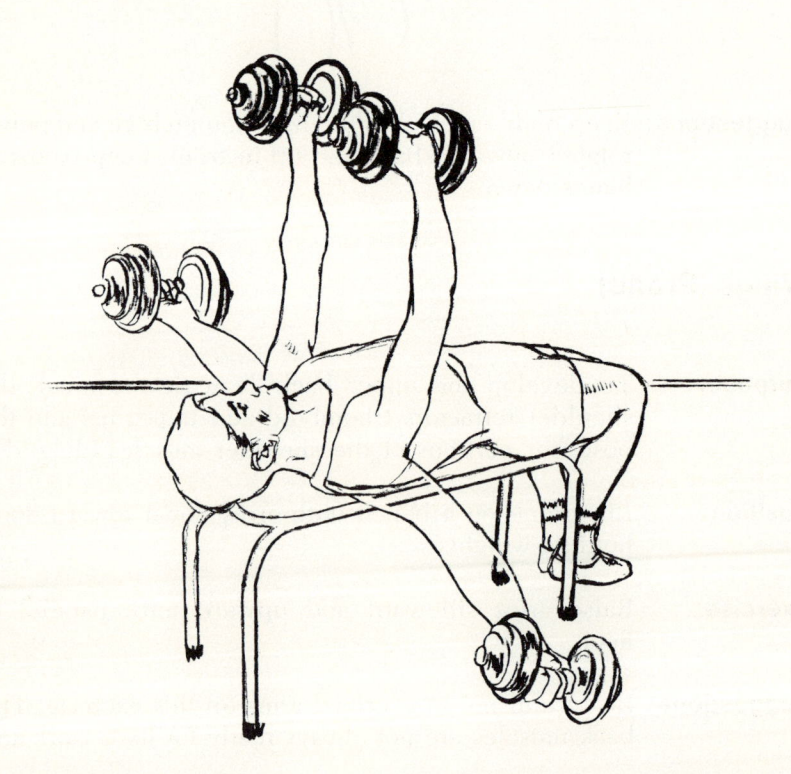

Purpose: To develop the anterior shoulder and chest muscles (the anterior deltoid, pectoralis major, coracobrachialis and serratus anterior).

Position: Lie on the back on a bench with the arms in a side horizontal position.

Exercise: Raise arms vertically above chest, keeping arms straight.

Suggestions: Keep the lower back flat to avoid undue strain.

Rowing

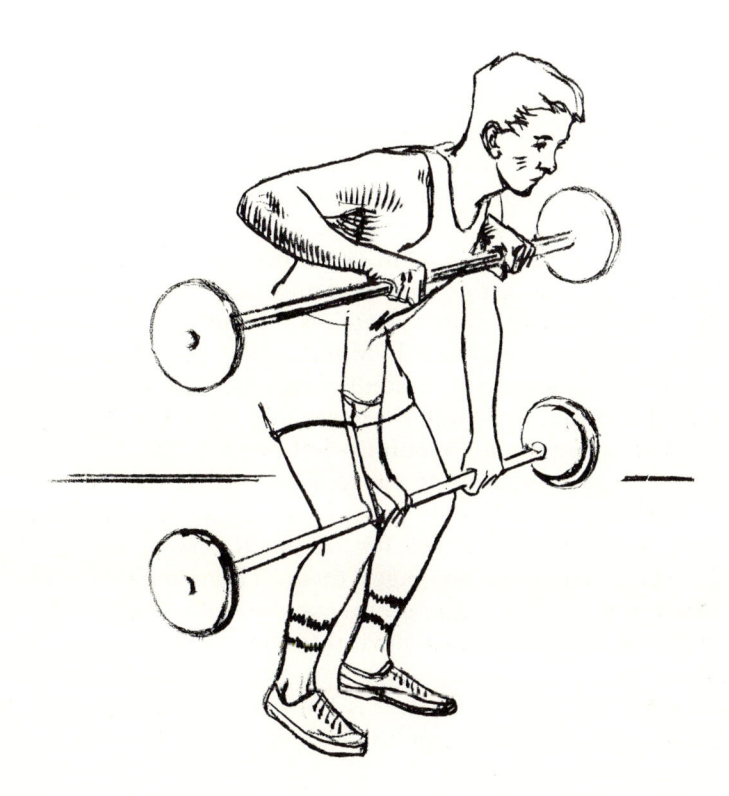

Purpose: To exercise the back (rhomboids), the shoulders (deltoids) and the front of the upper arms (biceps).

Position: Bend over at waist, upper body parallel to floor, weight at arms' length.

Exercise: Raise weight toward chest and pull in toward body. Push inward and downward while lowering weight.

Suggestions: When the hands are brought to the chest, pull shoulders back to exercise the upper back muscles. Anyone with back difficulty should not attempt this lift.

FLEXIBILITY EXERCISE

It is important to the athlete to develop a reasonable degree of flexibility, the full range of movement in a joint and the elasticity of the muscles that move it. The importance of flexibility to effective performance is particularly evident in such sports as wrestling, diving and hurdling, which require an extensive range of movement in a great many of the joints of the body. Flexibility is advantageous in other sports, also, although the need is less apparent. In running, for example, flexibility is needed in the hip and ankle joints to allow the runner to take a long stride without resistance from tight muscles.

Flexibility is developed by forcing the joint through an ever-widening range of movement. Two different methods of exercise may be employed to accomplish this: ballistic and static. Ballistic exercise refers to a movement of muscles made with such force that the momentum continues the movement beyond its normal range, thereby effecting a stretching of the opposing muscles. Static exercise refers to the holding of a position that stretches the muscles to their greatest possible length; the position is held for a short period of time.

Both methods appear to produce flexibility at approximately the same rate. However, the static exercises appear to be a better choice as stretching exercises for warm-up before a practice session. The ballistic exercises are likely to cause sore muscles. Static stretching tends to relieve soreness and requires less energy expenditure; hence, the athlete has more energy left for the practice session.

The static exercises on pages 69 to 71 are recommended for use in warming up. The entire group may be used, or a selection may be made of those that increase flexibility in the muscles most used in a particular sport.

When the position is taken, it is held for 30 to 60 seconds. Each exercise may be repeated three times, holding for 30 seconds with a rest interval of 10 seconds.

Lower Trunk Stretcher

Purpose: To increase the flexibility of the back flexor muscles.

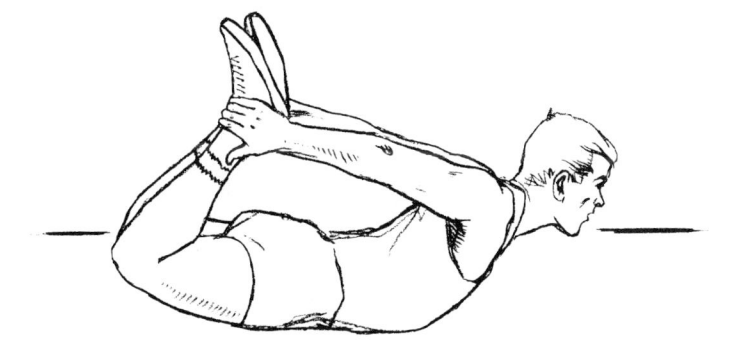

Position: Lie face down on the floor.

Exercise: Extend the arms behind to grasp the ankles and pull. Force the head back in the direction of the feet.

Upper Back Stretcher

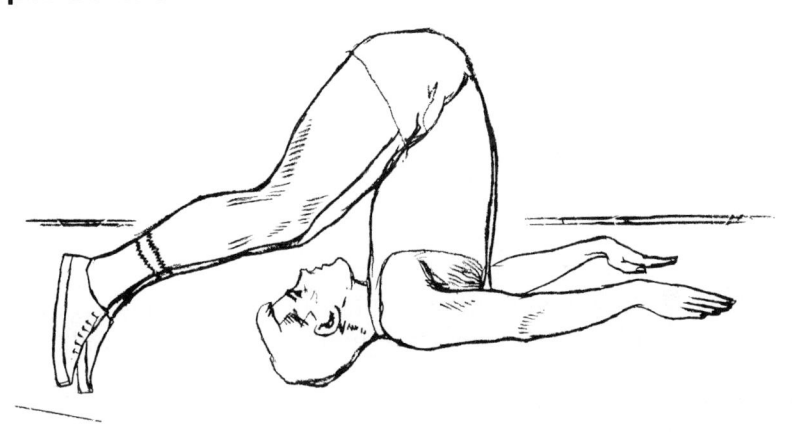

Purpose: To increase the flexibility of the back extensor muscles.

Position: Lie supine on the floor.

Exercise: Raise the legs up over the head and touch the toes to the floor. The hands and arms must remain flat on the floor.

Ankle Stretcher

Purpose: To increase the flexibility of the ankle flexor muscles.

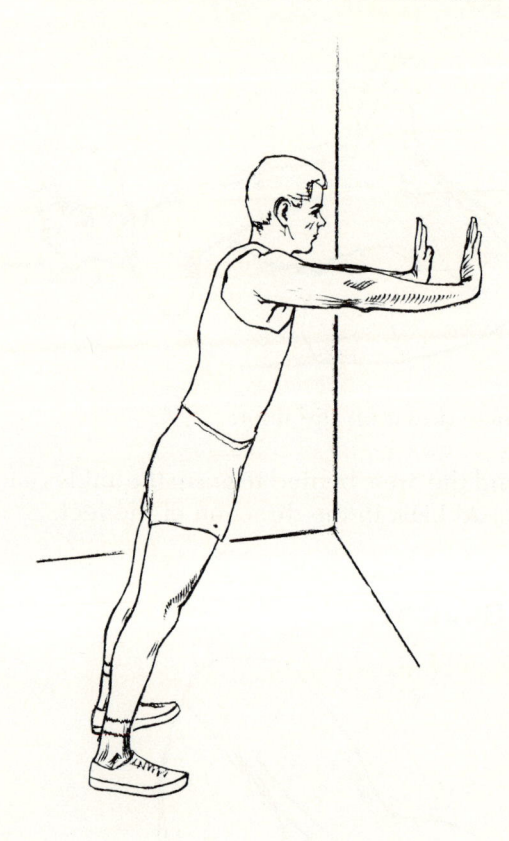

Position: Take a front leaning position, resting the hands against the wall, with the feet three to four feet from the wall.

Exercise: Keeping the body straight, lean toward the wall. The feet must remain parallel and flat on the floor.

Ankle Stretcher

Purpose: To increase the flexibility of the ankle extensor muscles.

Position: Take a sitting position with legs bent under the body and hips resting between ankles.

Exercise: Place the hands with palms down on the floor just behind the hips. Raise the knees from the floor as far as possible.

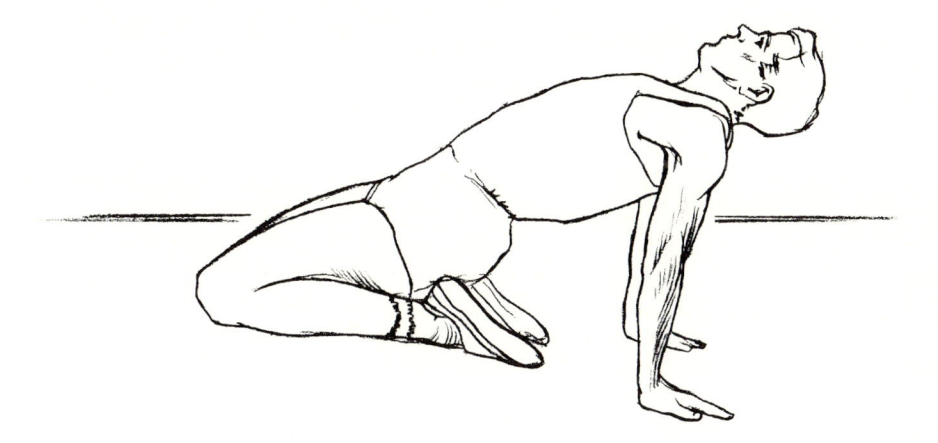

Shoulder Stretcher

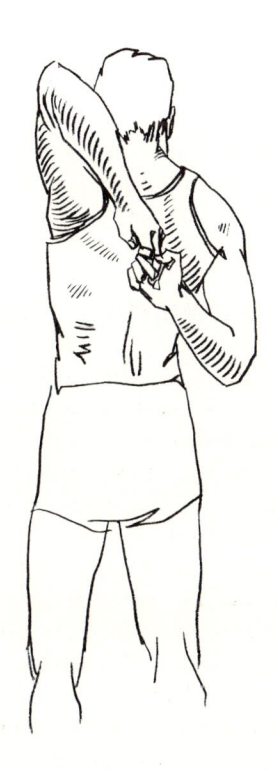

Purpose: To increase the flexibility of the shoulders.

Position: Stand upright.

Exercise: Bring the right hand to the upper back from above and the left hand from below and hook the fingers. Repeat reversing the hands.

Arm and Leg Stretcher

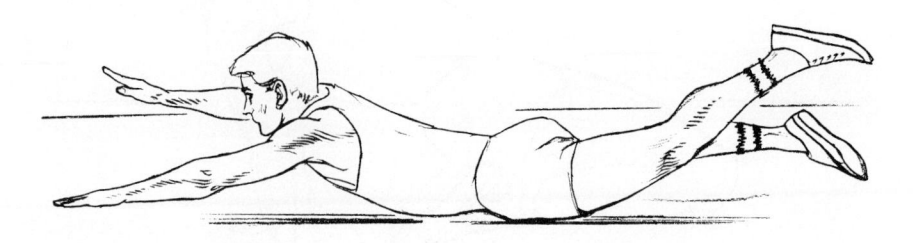

Purpose: To increase the flexibility of the arms and legs.

Position: Lie face down with the arms and legs extended.

Exercise: Raise the left arm and right leg simultaneously and then the right arm and left leg, alternately and in rapid succession.

PULLEY WEIGHT EXERCISE

Pulley weights utilize a pulley arrangement with attached weights to create resistance to pull exerted by the muscles of the arms and shoulders. The pulleys are attached at three levels, above the head, at chest height and near the floor, to produce different leverages for the exercise of different muscles. This makes possible a more complete workout for the muscles of the arms and shoulders than is possible in other forms of exercise. An additional advantage of the pulley weights is that the arm movements of a sport, such as a stroke in swimming or batting in baseball, may be simulated in an exercise and performed with complete confidence that the workout will contribute to the development of the muscles required by that particular action in the game situation.

If pulley weights are not available, shock cord, which is elastic, may be purchased at reasonable cost and attached to the wall at three levels to resemble the pulley weight arrangement. The exercise provided in this way is nearly identical to that of pulley weights.

The participant should continue the initial exercise until fatigued, note the number of repetitions accomplished and strive to increase this number in each successive workout. When improvement reaches a plateau, the amount of weight may be increased.

Overhead Exercise

Purpose: To develop the arm depressors (latissimus and pectoralis muscles).

Position: Stand with the back to the pulleys and the feet about eight inches from the wall. Grasp both handles of the overhead pulleys and lean back against the wall.

Exercise: Keeping the arms straight, pull forward and down to the hips. Return to the original position and repeat.

Suggestions: The pull down may also be done by moving the arms to the sides and then down, keeping the arms straight.

Floor Level Exercise

Purpose: To develop the flexors of the arm.

Position: Lie on the back with the feet toward the pulleys. Grasp both handles of the floor level pulleys with the palms up.

Exercise: With the elbows maintaining contact with the floor, bend the arms to raise the lower arms. Return to the original position and repeat.

Suggestions: Grasp the handles with the palms down to give exercise to the muscles that extend the wrists.

Floor Level Exercise

Purpose: To develop the strength of the shoulder abductors (deltoid muscles).

Position: Lie on the back with the feet toward pulleys. Grasp the handles of the floor level pulleys and hold the arms against the body.

Exercise: Keeping the arms straight, bring the arms to the side-horizontal position and return to the original position. Repeat.

Suggestions: Bring the arms to the front to stress the front portion of the shoulder (deltoid muscle).

Chest Level Exercise

Purpose: To develop the muscles of the chest (pectoralis) and the flexors of the arms.

Position: Stand, facing away from the pulleys, about three feet in front of the chest level pulleys. Grasp the handles and hold them out to the sides at shoulder height.

Exercise: Bring the hands forward and together. Return to the original position and repeat.

Chest Level Exercise

Purpose: To develop the shoulder muscles of the back (rhomboid, trapezius) and the extensors of the shoulder.

Position: Stand facing the pulleys about arms' distance from the wall. Grasp the handles of the chest level pulleys.

Exercise: Bring the arms back as far as possible, keeping them parallel to the floor.

UNIT IV

EVALUATION
THE YALE TESTS
A.A.H.P.E.R. TESTS
SIGMA DELTA PSI TEST

EVALUATION

The success of the conditioning program can be assessed by evaluating the amount of progress achieved over a period of time. A reliable evaluation requires a testing procedure in which the same factors are measured at periodic intervals. One of the most effective means of accomplishing this is to measure those components of physical fitness that are readily improved by a conditioning program. Among these components are: muscular strength and endurance, speed of movement, power and cardiorespiratory endurance.

Several batteries of tests that measure these components have been developed. One that has proved to be a highly effective measurement of the components of physical fitness is the Yale University Physical Fitness Battery, and it is recommended for use in determining the status of physical fitness and evaluating the success of the conditioning program. The battery includes the Vertical Jump, Pull-ups, Hand Grips, Dips or Push-ups, Broad Jump, Sit-ups and the Step Test. Measurements of height and weight are also included to give a more complete indication of the general physical condition. The norms for the test items listed on the following pages have been established on the results of tests of over 18,000 college men over a period of 26 years.

Another recommended physical fitness test battery is that developed by the American Association for Health, Physical Education and Recreation, known as the AAHPER Youth Fitness Test. The test items include: Pull-ups, Sit-ups, Shuttle Run, Standing Broad Jump, 50 Yard Dash, Softball Throw and 600 Yard Run-walk. This battery may be used to advantage both for measuring progress and for exercise in a conditioning program.

Supplementary test items may be added to any battery of tests or items may be subtracted, depending upon the kind of measurement desired. Items may be chosen to give additional evaluation of physical fitness as related to specific sports. In a conditoning program aimed at improving ability in a specific sport, test items that measure factors basic to the ability would, of course, be a necessary addition to the general physical fitness battery. For example, if leg strength is one of the elements that the sport demands, the leg lift measurement should be included in the tests.

One of the finest all-around tests in sports skills and fitness is that used by a national physical education fraternity, Sigma Delta Psi. This society was founded at the University of Indiana in 1912 and incorporated in 1930. Membership is open to college students in good academic standing and eligible for competition in varsity athletics who have successfully passed the various tests in the presence of a faculty member or a member of the college staff on the test committee. Membership in this organization is for the athlete the equivalent of Phi Beta Kappa membership for the high-ranking scholar. Among the skills tested are running, jumping, hurdling, throwing, swimming, tumbling and climbing.

Taking the Tests

The battery of tests should be taken at the start of the conditioning program for a complete record of the physical fitness status with which to compare later test results in order to assess the progress made. The amount of improvement that will be evidenced will depend upon the amount of exercise and work demanded of the body by the conditioning program and the amount of time and effort given to the program. Generally speaking, no appreciable changes in the level of physical fitness will be noted in less than three or four weeks of regular systematic exercising. Therefore, a test to determine progress may wait until after the first month of conditioning. In college physical education programs, the testing is usually made twice a semester, once at the beginning of the semester and once at the end.

It is suggested that you keep a record of scores on the test items on the chart provided on page 77.

Height

The height is taken in stocking or bare feet on a platform which is part of the weighing device. The height scale is also arranged for individuals who are measured wearing shoes. Care should be taken

Personal Fitness Record

Name								
Age		Years		Months		Days		
Height (ins.)								
Weight (lbs.)								
Date								
Class								
Test		No. 1		No. 2		No. 3		No. 4
	Date →							
Grips		RT.	LT.	RT.	LT.	RT.	LT.	RT. LT.
Vertical Jump								
Chins (Bent arm hang)								
Sit-up								
Standing Broad Jump								
Fence Vault								
Push Ups								
Dips								
Leg Lifts								
Back Lifts								
Push (Pectorals)								
Pull (Retractors)								

*AAHPER TEST

Test		Score	Per Cent	Score	Per Cent	Score	Per Cent
	Date →						
Pull-up							
Arm Hang							
Sit-up							
Shuttle Run							
Standing Broad Jump							
50 Yard Dash							
Softball Throw							
		Pulse	Total	Pulse	Total	Pulse	Total
Brouha Step Test	1.						
	2.		Index ↓		Index ↓		Index ↓
	3.						

*Use the appropriate classification tables in the AAHPER Youth Fitness Test Manual to find your percentile scores.

to see that the measure arm, which touches the top of head, is parallel to the floor.

The subject stands "tall," with the abdomen in, the head erect and the back straight. The measurement is recorded in eighths or tenths of inches. The old device of tacking a yardstick on the back of a door or on a door jamb and using it to measure height is also useful for this test. In a class situation in which measurement is taken infrequently, accuracy should be stressed and care should be taken to eliminate variables insofar as possible.

Weight

The weight is usually recorded along with the height. The accuracy of modern scales has improved considerably. The weight should be taken, when convenient, without clothing.

Height and weight measurements may be compared with figures in Table 1 (Unit II, page 8) and used for future reference in determining gain or loss of weight resulting from exercise and change in diet. Measurement of the high jump performance of the Sigma Delta Psi tests is based on height and weight classification. In the same battery of tests, body weight is used to determine distance ratings for the shot put.

THE YALE TESTS

Hand Grips

Purpose: To measure the gripping strength of the hands, which is dependent in large part upon lower arm strength. The test gives a good indication of general motor fitness.

Equipment: Hand dynamometer.

Position: Place the dynamometer across the palm of the hand with the fingers around it and the dial facing the palm of the hand.

Procedure: Squeeze the dynamometer as hard as possible. Movements of the body are not allowed. Two attempts are made with each hand; the higher reading for each hand is the score.

Suggestions: Care should be taken to remove the dynamometer from the hand without moving it from side to side, which may move the needle and disqualify the reading. Chalk or resin may be used on the hands if they are wet with perspiration.

Rating:

	Right hand	*Left hand*
Desirable score	140	130
Poor	Below 100	90
Fair	100 to 120	91 to 110
Good	121 to 140	111 to 135
Excellent	Over 140	135

Vertical Jump

Purpose: To measure the explosive leg strength.

Equipment: A measuring board, such as a piece of masonite painted black, or a large flat wall surface marked with parallel lines one inch apart for (a) measuring the reaching height and (b) the jumping height.

Position: Stand with toes against and facing the measuring board.

Procedure: Reach with both hands and touch a point on the board as high as possible without straining. Then jump, as in the basketball center jump, and touch the board at the highest point. The distance between the standing reach and jumping touch is then measured for the score.

Suggestions: Two or three jumps are allowed. No stepping or running is permitted. Experimenting with one or the other arm for the jump-touch may be helpful. Chalk on the fingertips aids in the marking of the touch.

Rating:

	Desirable score	20 inches
	Poor	15 inches or less
	Fair	16 to 17 inches
	Good	18 to 20 inches
	Excellent	20 inches or more

Sit-ups

Purpose: To measure the endurance of the hip flexors when the legs are straight or of the abdominal muscles when the knees are bent.

Equipment: A bench, stall bar or a second person to hold the feet or ankles.

Position: Take a supine position on the floor with the hands behind the head, bend the knees, and have the feet held by a partner or anchor them under a stall bar or bench.

Procedure: Raise the trunk to a sitting position, and with each sit-up twist alternately left and right. As you twist, touch the elbow to the opposite knee. Each return to the original position is counted as one sit-up.

Suggestions: The knees are bent to allow the abdominal muscles to come into play. When the knees are straight, the abdominal action is minimal and the hip flexors are stressed.

Rating:
Desirable number		60
Poor		0 to 20
Fair		21 to 40
Good		41 to 60
Excellent		Over 60

Pull-ups

Purpose: To measure the strength of the shoulder girdle and of the arms in their ability to depress the shoulder and lift the body weight.

Equipment: A suitable bar, high enough so that the feet are off the floor when in a hanging position.

Position: Grasp bar with palms of hands forward. Assume a hanging position, arms and legs extended.

Procedure: Pull the body up toward the bar until the chin is over the bar. Lower slowly and assume the original position. Knees may be bent but must be kept bent and the body must not swing. The number of complete pull-ups is the score.

Suggestions: A second person may help to prevent swinging of the body.

Rating:
Desirable number		8
Poor		0 to 3
Fair		4 to 5
Good		6 to 8
Excellent		Over 8

Standing Broad Jump

Purpose: To measure the explosive leg strength.

Equipment: A mat made of nonslip material.

Position: Stand with feet comfortably apart and toes behind take-off line.

Procedure: Swing arms forcefully forward and upward; take off from the balls of the feet. The landing is made on the heels with the feet parallel. The distance jumped is measured from the take-off line to the heel or any part of the body that touches the ground nearest the take-off line. Three trials are allowed. Record the best of the three trials in feet and inches.

Suggestions: Allow one practice jump. Be sure the area is clear beyond the landing point.

Rating:

Desirable distance	90 inches
Poor	60 to 70 inches
Fair	71 to 80 inches
Good	81 to 90 inches
Excellent	Over 90 inches

Dips

Purpose: To measure the extension strength of the arms in lifting the body. Dips are more objectively performed and higher in validity of strength measurement than push-ups.

Equipment: A parallel bar or wall bracket with arms about shoulder width, high enough so the feet are off the floor.

Position: Assume a cross-rest position on the parallel bars with arms straight.

Procedure: Lower the trunk to a point at which the elbow joints form right angles or less. Raise the trunk by pushing up until the arms are again fully extended. Each return to this position shall be counted as one dip.

Suggestions: To insure that the correct procedure is followed the scorer may use his hand to mark the height. The performer's shoulder must touch.

Rating: Desirable number   10
           Poor   0 to 4
           Fair   5 to 7
           Good   8 to 10
           Excellent   Over 10

Push-ups

Purpose: To measure the extension strength of the arms. Push-ups are an excellent exercise as well as a test that can be used in place of dips.

Equipment: No equipment is needed. Any flat surface is adequate.

Position: Lie prone, body straight, hands flat on the floor at the level of the shoulders, toes extended to support feet and body.

Procedure: Push the body up from the floor, keeping the body straight, to a fully extended arm position. Lower the body until right angles are formed at the elbows. Each time the return to the straight position is made, it shall count as one push-up.

Rating: Desirable number   30
           Poor   0 to 15
           Fair   16 to 20
           Good   21 to 30
           Excellent   Over 30

Fence Vault (Bar Vault)

Purpose: To measure the strength of the legs when coordinating with the arms in a vaulting action.

Equipment: A crossbar four feet, six inches high, which can be moved to various heights, and a mat for protection of the feet and legs in landing.

Position: Stand, facing the bar. Place the hands on the bar shoulders' width apart.

Procedure: Jump to a straight arm position over the bar, lift the legs (which are kept together) over the bar. Push with hands and let go of the hand nearer the side to which the legs are carried. When the body is clear over one hand, let go with the second hand and land facing the same direction as in the start; this is considered a passing score.

Suggestions: If the feet hit the bar, hold on to the bar to keep from falling heavily to the floor. Two or three trials are allowed. No stepping or running is permitted and no part of the body (except the hands) may touch the bar. It is desirable to use a spotter.

Rating:

Desirable height	4 feet, 6 inches
Poor	3 feet 8 inches to 4 feet 2 inches
Fair	4 feet 3 inches to 4 feet 6 inches
Good	4 feet 7 inches to 4 feet 8 inches
Excellent	Over 4 feet 8 inches

The Step Test*

Purpose: To measure endurance of the cardiorespiratory system.

Equipment: A bench or stool (20 inches high), a stop watch and a metronome or a recording tape to keep the rhythm for the five-minute test.

Position: Stand on the floor facing the bench or stool.

Procedure: Step up on the bench with one foot and bring the other foot up until both legs are straight at the knees. Return to the original position on the floor in the same manner. This is done 30 times a minute in rhythm for a period of five minutes. A good cadence is: up, step—down, step.

Following the five minutes of exercise, one minute rest is taken in a sitting position. Three pulse counts of 30 seconds duration each are taken by a second person or by yourself at the carotid artery of the neck, at six minutes, at seven minutes and at eight minutes. These three pulse counts are totaled and called the recovery rate.

---

*Brouha, Lucien. The step test. The Research Quarterly, volume 14, number 1. March, 1943.

If you fail to complete five minutes of the step test, no pulse is taken and no score registered. The number of minutes performed, however, is noted and the test can be taken periodically until the five-minute minimum can be performed.

Rating: Table 2 below will indicate your fitness index. Above 90 is superior or excellent and below 50 poor.

Table 2. Recovery Table for the Step Test

Duration of Exercise: 300 Seconds

Recovery Rate	Fitness Index	Recovery Rate	Fitness Index	Recovery Rate	Fitness Index	Recovery Rate	Fitness Index
150	100.0	180	83.4	210	71.4	240	62.6
151	99.3	181	83.0	211	71.2	241	62.3
152	98.7	182	82.5	212	70.7	242	62.0
153	98.0	183	82.0	213	70.4	243	61.8
154	97.4	184	81.5	214	70.1	244	61.5
155	96.8	185	81.1	215	69.7	245	61.3
156	96.2	186	80.7	216	69.4	246	61.0
157	95.6	187	80.2	217	69.1	247	60.8
158	95.0	188	79.8	218	68.8	248	60.5
159	94.3	189	79.4	219	68.5	249	60.3
160	93.8	190	78.9	220	68.2	250	60.0
161	93.2	191	78.6	221	67.9	251	59.8
162	92.6	192	78.1	222	67.6	252	59.6
163	92.0	193	77.7	223	67.3	253	59.3
164	91.5	194	77.3	224	67.0	254	59.1
165	90.9	195	77.0	225	66.7	255	58.8
166	90.4	196	76.5	226	66.4	256	58.6
167	89.9	197	76.2	227	66.1	257	58.4
168	89.4	198	75.8	228	65.8	258	58.2
169	88.8	199	75.4	229	65.5	259	57.9
170	88.3	200	75.0	230	65.3	260	57.7
171	87.8	201	74.6	231	64.9	261	57.5
172	87.2	202	74.3	232	64.7	262	57.3
173	86.8	203	73.9	233	64.4	263	57.0
174	86.2	204	73.5	234	64.1	264	56.9
175	85.7	205	73.2	235	63.9	265	56.6
176	85.3	206	72.9	236	63.6	266	56.4
177	84.7	207	72.4	237	63.4	267	56.2
178	84.3	208	72.1	238	63.1	268	55.9
179	83.8	209	71.9	239	62.8	269	55.7

Classification or Rating of Physical Fitness Step Test

Below 55	Poor physical condition
55-64	Low average to fair
65-80	Average to good
80-90	Good to very good
Above 90	Superior, excellent

AAHPER TESTS*

Pull-up

As explained in the Yale Test, page 78.

Rating:
	Desirable number	9
	Poor	0 to 3
	Fair	4 to 5
	Good	6 to 8
	Excellent	Over 9

Sit-ups

As explained in the Yale Test (page 79), with the exception that the legs may be kept straight.

Rating:
	Desirable number	61
	Poor	Less than 40
	Fair	41 to 50
	Good	51 to 60
	Excellent	Over 61

Shuttle Run

Purpose: To measure speed and agility in running.

Equipment: A stop watch, two blocks of wood (2 in. × 2 in. × 4 in.) and two parallel lines marked on the floor 30 feet apart.

Procedure: Place the blocks behind one of the lines. Start from behind the other line. On the signal to go run to the blocks, pick one up, run back to the starting line and place the block behind the line; then run back and pick up the second block and carry it back across the starting line. Two trials, with rest between, are allowed.

Rating: Record the better of the two trials to the nearest tenth of a second.
Desirable time   9.2 seconds

---

*For percentile score for men and women see *AAHPER Test Manual*, 1201 16th St. NW, Washington, D.C.

Poor	10.0 to 18 seconds
Fair	9.4 to 9.9 seconds
Good	8.3 to 9.3 seconds
Excellent	Less than 8.3 seconds

Standing Broad Jump

As explained in Yale Test, page 80. Score is measured in inches.

Rating:
	Desirable distance	90 inches
	Poor	Less than 80 inches
	Fair	71 to 80 inches
	Good	81 to 90 inches
	Excellent	Over 90 inches

50-yard Dash

Purpose: To measure the speed of movement in running.

Equipment: Stop watch; 50 yard running area with start and finish lines clearly marked.

Procedure: On the command to go, run as fast as possible to the finish line. The score is the time it takes to run the distance, measured in tenths of seconds.

Rating:
	Desirable time	61 seconds
	Poor	69 seconds or over
	Fair	66 to 69 seconds
	Good	62 to 65 seconds
	Excellent	Less than 62 seconds

Softball Throw for Distance

Purpose: To measure the arm strength and coordination (throwing ability) by the distance the softball can be thrown.

Equipment: Softball (12 inch), small metal or wooden stakes and tape measure. A football field marked in conventional fashion (five-yard intervals) makes an ideal area for this test. A restraining area is designated by marking two parallel lines six feet apart.

Procedure: Throw the ball while remaining within the parallel lines. Only an overhand throw may be used; three throws are allowed. The distance measured is the distance from the point of landing to the nearest point on the restraining line. Record the best of three throws to the nearest foot.

Rating:
Desirable distance	220 feet
Poor	64 to 167 feet
Fair	168 to 193 feet
Good	194 to 220 feet
Excellent	Over 220 feet

600 Yard Run-Walk

Purpose: To measure speed and endurance in distance running.

Equipment: Running area and stop watch.

Procedure: At the signal "Go!" begin running the 600-yard distance. Walking is permitted, but the distance must be covered in the shortest possible time. The time is recorded in minutes and seconds.

Rating:
Desirable time	1:43
Poor	Over 2 minutes
Fair	1:50 to 2:00
Good	1:44 to 1:49
Excellent	Less than 1:44

THE SIGMA DELTA PSI TEST*

Test Items	Minimum Standard
1. 100-yard dash	11.6 seconds
2. 120-yard low hurdles	16 seconds
3. Running high jump	Ht.-wt. classification
4. Running broad jump	17 feet
5. 16-pound shot put	30 ft. or wt. classification
6. 20-foot rope climb	12 seconds
or golf test	4 out of 5 shots

---

*Address correspondence about the test to Joseph Picard, 108 B Men's Gymnasium, University of Arizona, Tucson.

7. Baseball throw	250 feet
or javelin throw	130 feet
8. Football punt	120 feet
9. 100-yard swim	1 minute 45 seconds
10. 1-mile run	6 minutes
11. Front handspring	Land on feet with good form
12. Handstand	10 seconds
or bowling test	160 ave. for 3 games
13. Fence vault	Chin high
14. Good posture	B standard of the Harvard Body Mechanics Posture Charts†
15. Scholarship	Eligible for varsity competition

When a student has passed the above tests the faculty adviser may submit his record to the national chapter for consideration for membership. The record should show the date tests were passed and the initials of the examiner.

The following excerpts from the Sigma Delta Psi Consitution are quoted for information about the fraternity and about the administration of the test items.

Purpose

The object of the society shall be to promote physical, mental, and moral development of college students.
1. Chapters of this society may be installed at any accredited college in the United States offering a four-year course of study.

    Membership is open to college students in good academic standing who have successfully passed the various tests in the presence of a faculty member or authorized person.
2. All male students in colleges in the United States shall be eligible to membership. The Physical Education Director certifies fitness of candidate.
3. Requirements for Full Membership:

    Section 1. For admission to full membership a student shall successfully attain the marks set opposite the following events in the presence of at least one faculty member or the authorized director of the certification committee.

    Section 2. The Director of Physical Education shall certify to the physical fitness of a candidate before being allowed to attempt any of the tests.

    Section 3. A candidate shall be permitted to attempt only

---

†Department of Hygiene and Physical Education, Harvard University, Cambridge, Mass.

three tests on a single day. Only three official trials shall be permitted in any test during a single day.

Section 4. A candidate may attempt to qualify in Sigma Delta Psi any time while a student or as an alumnus from his institution.

Section 5.
- a. Test No. 2. Five standard low hurdles shall be used to a flight, placed twenty yards apart. The test to be valid, all hurdles must remain upright from their bases.
- b. Test No. 5. Thirty feet to be requirement for a man of 160 pounds or over, the requirement to be scaled down in accordance with the following proportion for candidate's weight as 30 feet is to the requirement.
- c. Test No. 6. The candidates shall start from a sitting position on the floor and climb rope without use of legs. Legs may be used in the descent.
- d. Test No. 12. The candidate shall not be compelled to remain stationary during the test, neither shall he be allowed to advance or retreat more than three feet in any direction.
- e. Test No. 14. The candidate shall be required to pass the B Standard of the Harvard Body Mechanics Posture Chart. These charts will be furnished all local chapters. The Committee or Director should observe the candidate's posture when he is not aware of the fact.
- f. Test numbers 1, 2, 5, 6, 7, and 8 shall be attempted cross-wise or into the wind to be accepted by the Director of Committee on Certification.
- g. The National Collegiate Rules for the various activities of the tests are the accepted standards.

4. Substitution: A candidate who has won the varsity letter or an intramural championship in any sport may substitute this letter for any one requirement in Sigma Delta Psi, except swimming. A substitution may be made but once for one sport; for example, the candidate may substitute the football award but once, even though he plays on the varsity team three years. The privilege of substitution of varsity letters is limited to two official varsity sports and one intramural championship.

An intramural championship shall consist of at least sixteen competitors to a tournament and at least eight men to a division, class, etc.

UNIT V

TRAINING FOR ENDURANCE
RUNNING AND JOGGING
SWIMMING
STAIR CLIMBING
BENCH STEPPING
BICYCLING
ROWING

TRAINING FOR ENDURANCE

Any conditioning program should include some type of activity that provides a workout for the heart and the lungs. As pointed out in the discussion of the benefits of exercise, increasing the demands on these organs will help to develop cardiorespiratory endurance, which is the ability of the body cells to obtain and use oxygen and to rid the body of carbon dioxide; the heart and lungs play important roles in this process. When greater than customary demands for oxygen occur as the result of activity requiring great endurance, the functioning of the heart and the lungs improves. Regular and continued participation in activities such as jogging, running, swimming and bicycling will provide the kind of workout needed to develop cardiorespiratory endurance. Rowing, stair climbing and bench stepping are other possibilities that are equally good but less popular.

RUNNING AND JOGGING

In most respects running and jogging are similar and each provides the same kind of workout. The chief difference between the two appears to be in the motivation of those who run and those who jog. The runner is motivated by the challenge of competition; his interest in running centers on competing against an opponent or against his own previous record. The jogger, on the other hand, is motivated by the joy of running and his recognition of the physiological values that accrue. Probably everyone who is either a runner or a jogger at some time or another both runs and jogs but, as a general rule he is predominantly one or the other. Runners in track events do, of course, use jogging as a method of warming up before intensive practice or competitive races.

Good form in either jogging or running is important for ease of movement, unrestricted breathing and prevention of muscular soreness. There are two distinct running forms: the sprint form and the long distance running form. The latter is also used in jogging.

The extent of participation in any activity is dependent upon the pleasure one derives from it. Running and jogging will be more pleasant if some consideration is given to the kind of clothing and shoes worn for the activity. The clothing should be comfortably loose so there will be no binding or chafing, and it should be light enough to be comfortable when the body becomes heated from running. It is desirable to have several sets of appropriate workout clothes so that one clean, fresh outfit will always be available when others are being laundered. Lightweight but sturdy shoes or sneakers are necessary for running comfort. The shoes should fit neither too snugly nor too loosely. Socks should be worn to absorb the perspiration and to aid in the prevention of blisters; to be effective, the socks must be clean.

Any signs of blisters or irritations of the feet or irritations of the crotch, underarms or elsewhere on the body should be promptly checked as to cause and treated. Further workouts should cease until the source of the trouble has been eliminated.

Sprint Form

In the sprints the rear leg exerts great force to drive the body forward. As the leg completes its drive, it is brought forward with the heel carried high under the hip. The thigh swings forward parallel to the ground; the knee is bent as the thigh is swung forward. The knee is then extended, and the other leg (now the rear leg) exerts force to drive the body up and forward. At this instant there is no contact with the ground. The knee of the forward leg is bent very slightly. Contact with the ground is made with the toes straight ahead.

The arms are swung forward and backward from the shoulder. When the leg is brought forward, the opposite arm is brought forward. The elbow is bent at a 90 degree angle. Care should be taken not to swing the arms in front of the chest while running for this will cause the body to twist or wobble from side to side.

At full speed the body is carried at a slight angle. The head should be held in a natural position.

Long Distance and Jogging Form

In jogging or running long distances, a much shorter stride is used, and much less force will be exerted by the back foot. The trunk angle is greater than in sprinting. The arm action is less vigorous since the leg force is less. The arm angle may be as great as 125 degrees.

The stride should be smooth and rhythmic. The foot should land on the ground, toes pointing straight ahead, with a heel-ball effect. This is accomplished by rocking the foot over onto the ball after the heel has contacted the ground. In this way the shock of the landing is absorbed more nearly by the whole foot.

Pace

How fast or how far should one run? The speed depends upon the distance and the distance upon the speed. This relationship of speed and distance is involved in what track men call pace. Pace is a specific rate of movement for any given distance; for example, to run a four-minute mile, the runner would have to run at a rate that would enable him to cover each quarter mile in one minute. If he failed to keep the pace in one quarter, he would have to increase his pace to make up the lost time in the next quarter. To break it down further, he would have to run each 110 yards in 15 seconds. Experienced track athletes become expert at gauging pace and can determine readily how much energy and effort to expend during each interval of the total distance to achieve maximum results. Some runners carry a stop watch with them while running to insure a correct pace. Others rely on a signal from their coach at a certain point in the course.

For the beginning jogger or runner, pace is not important. The important measure at this stage is how far he can run. Depending upon the general condition of the runner's body, the achievable distance at first might range between 100 yards and 2 miles. Except when training for a particular event, there is little need to run or jog more than two miles for general conditioning purposes. A good standard distance for most beginners is one mile.

A good technique in the early stages is to run a short distance, then walk a short distance, and repeat the activities. As the body becomes better conditioned, the amount of walking is decreased. It is suggested that no rest periods of complete inactivity be taken during the run as the walking periods will provide sufficient rest. If any nausea occurs, the runner should stop for that day.

Once a mile can be run without difficulty, the element of time becomes important. Following a pace schedule is then the answer to the speed one should run. The following procedure is suggested:

1. Determine how long it takes you to run one mile on a standard track or on the open road.

2. Divide your best time into 16 parts. Each part represents your time for 110 yards.
3. Establish intervals of 110 yards on your running route.
4. Now try to run your mile, keeping approximately the same speed for each 110 yards; for example, if you ran your mile in eight minutes, you would have averaged 30 seconds for each 110 yards. See if you can consciously do the same by checking a watch or clock. Once you can, a feeling for pace has been established.
5. The final step in the procedure is to increase the speed gradually at intervals of 110 yards. If you run one second faster each third 110, you will have cut five seconds from your original time. By cutting seconds off gradually, you will eventually reach a period of constancy. This may be either a plateau, which is temporary, or may measure the limit of your capabilities.

These procedures have been suggested for several general reasons. In the first place, one mile is a standard measure which can be easily divided into halves, quarters, eighths or sixteenths. It is a long enough distance to develop endurance, yet not prohibitive in length to the novice. The division into sixteenths (110 yards) has been suggested, particularly for the beginner, because it is easier to run and walk short distances. Those in good condition may use a quarter mile as the interval for establishing a standard pace.

When the track being used is not a standard measure but has been measured for the number of laps per mile, it may be simpler to use each lap as a unit of measure for setting pace.

The pace chart

The Pace Chart (Table 3) is useful in establishing a basic running program. It is gauged so that an individual can determine how many seconds it will take him to run, at 110-yard intervals, any distance up to one mile. It will also tell him what his time should be at any given distance. Beginning on the extreme left at the top of the chart opposite 110 yards is the figure 30, indicating 30 seconds. By following down in that column, you can see that it takes 60 seconds to run 220 yards, one minute and 30 seconds to run 330 yards, etc., up to eight minutes to run 1760 yards (one mile). The top figure in each column indicates the number of seconds in which one must run each 110 yards to achieve the time given at the bottom of the column for one mile. The times in the top columns run from left to right in descending order to the final column, which indicates that 15-second intervals for each 100 yards are necessary to run a four-minute mile.

It is obviously not feasible to run every lap in the exact same time

Table 3. Pace Chart

Distance in Yards	Time in Seconds								
110	:30	:28	:26	:24	:22	:20	:18	:16	:15
220	1:00	:56	:52	:48	:44	:40	:36	:32	:30
330	1:30	1:24	1:18	1:12	1:06	1:00	:54	:48	:45
440	2:00	1:52	1:44	1:36	1:28	1:20	1:12	1:04	1:00
550	2:30	2:20	2:10	2:00	1:50	1:40	1:30	1:20	1:15
660	3:00	2:48	2:36	2:24	2:12	2:00	1:48	1:36	1:30
770	3:30	3:16	3:02	2:48	2:34	2:20	2:06	1:52	1:45
880	4:00	3:44	3:28	3:12	2:56	2:40	2:24	2:08	2:00
990	4:30	4:12	3:54	3:36	3:18	3:00	2:42	2:24	2:15
1100	5:00	4:40	4:20	4:00	3:40	3:20	3:00	2:40	2.30
1210	5:30	5:08	4:46	4:24	4:02	3:40	3:18	2:56	2:45
1320	6:00	5:36	5:12	4:48	4:24	4:00	3:36	3:12	3:00
1430	6:30	6:04	5:38	5:12	4:46	4:20	3:54	3:28	3:15
1540	7:00	6:32	6:04	5:36	5:08	4:40	4:12	3:44	3:30
1650	7:30	7:00	6:30	6:00	5:30	5:00	4:30	4:00	3:45
1760	8:00	7:28	6:56	6:24	5:52	5:20	4:48	4:16	4:00

unless one is expert at pacing. For the novice, training for pace can be made easier by looking at a watch or clock and slowing down or speeding up, whichever is necessary, to reach a given point at a given time.

Some people prefer running a given distance at different paces, such as covering the first 200 yards at a fast rate of speed, and then running a steady race until the last 100 yards, when a sprint is made to the finish line. Many combinations are possible, and careful figuring of time can make what is usually an ordinary workout into a real challenge. Fading, or forced slowing down at the end of a run, is indicative of too fast a pace at the beginning or middle third of the distance to be run.

Interval Training

The general idea of interval training is to apply a constant amount of pressure with alternate periods of rest. A simple example is: ten 50-yard sprints, with one-minute rests between each 50 yards; follow this with five 100-yard sprints with two-minute rest periods in between, three series of 220 yards with three minutes rest, and two quarter-mile runs with a three-minute rest between. The term *rest* in interval training does not mean to stop moving entirely but, rather, to continue at a slower pace or walk.

The duration of the workout may be from 30 minutes to one hour or more. In 30-minute sessions a participant will cover (running and walking) a distance of three miles, more or less, while in a one-hour session he would come close to covering six miles. Some of the great runners have been known to run as much as 20 miles in interval training. Beginners will be amazed at the amount of work that can be accomplished using this method.

SWIMMING

Swimming is being used increasingly as a means of general body conditioning, particularly to improve cardiorespiratory endurance. The frequency with which it is used is attributable both to the great popularity of swimming with all age groups and to the increased number of indoor facilities available that make it possible to swim all year.

In swimming for conditioning, any stroke may be used. The crawl is used most frequently simply because it is the stroke most swimmers know. It is also a stroke that places a great demand upon the cardiorespiratory function of the body. However, if other strokes, especially the back stroke, are employed during the workout, a more complete workout for the body is provided.

Like the other endurance-building activities described in this unit, swimming may be participated in at a relatively leisurely pace or at a considerable rate of speed. The greater the speed, the greater the demands upon the body and the faster the rate of improvement in cardiorespiratory endurance.

For the beginner in a swimming program for conditioning, the first workouts should be continued only to the point of mild fatigue. The swimmer should note the distance he was able to swim and try to increase it in subsequent workouts. Gradual increase should occur as endurance improves.

Interval Training

When the swimmer is in good condition, he may begin interval training. Interval training in swimming is based on the same physiological principle as interval training in running, described previously. In this type of training, a specified distance is swum in a specific amount of time. A short rest is taken before the same distance is swum again in the same amount of time. The procedure is repeated several times; each time the demands on the swimmer are greater because he must overcome the fatigue factor to swim the distance in the same amount of time. The number of repetitions may be increased, the speed of swimming the repetitions may be increased or the time interval for recovery may be decreased to place a greater work load on the swimmer.

STAIR CLIMBING

An activity seldom used but extremely beneficial for developing cardiorespiratory endurance is stair climbing. Since it is the climbing up rather than the stepping down that creates the desired workout, long flights of stairs are more suitable for this activity.

Stairs are, in a sense, hills; and as many marathoners have said, "It's the hills that wear you down." Climbing is far more taxing on the circulatory system than jogging, and discretion must be used by each participant as to the amount of activity. When a very vigorous workout is desired, running up the stairs may replace walking.

The activity also develops the strength and endurance of the leg muscles. The knees should be straightened with each step in order to achieve maximum benefit in developing leg strength.

BENCH STEPPING

Stepping up on and down from a bench is another little-used but beneficial activity for developing the heart and lungs and also the legs. A bench or chair 20 inches high is used. A period of five minutes at a speed of 30 times per minute is sufficient for an average session with this particular exercise. However, longer periods can be endured with beneficial results when you become conditioned to it. Again, as in stair climbing, the legs should be fully extended up on the bench in order to get the most out of the exercise.

BICYCLING

Bicycling is in a sense very much like running. However, the differences can create many variables. The cyclist can coast downhill, whereas the runner must continue his leg movements. Sitting on a seat also eliminates much of the arm, shoulder and hip action involved in running. On the other hand, cycling is much more difficult going uphill than running, which can be reduced to a slow jog.

For the beginner, a safe level area is ideal for becoming familiar with the mechanics of movement involved and to begin conditioning. For endurance development, traveling uphill is a must. It usually is good practice to retrace the route in order to receive the benefit from traveling over the hills even though the action is reversed. For top effort, extremely hilly country should be chosen. When it seems that there are no more hills to conquer, the element of speed can be injected, as in running. There are obvious dangers in speed cycling, and great care should be exercised in selecting a safe place for the activity.

ROWING

Rowing can be an exhausting activity, producing great strain and fatigue. It can also be a pleasurable pastime. From the standpoint of developing endurance, a systematic approach is necessary, and regular, frequent practice sessions must be adhered to. One session per week of this activity could hardly qualify as being beneficial, as the soreness developed in one practice would only begin all over again in the next workout. Rowing endurance is usually developed by simply rowing longer distances at an increasingly faster pace.

UNIT VI

CONDITIONING FOR SPORTS
SPECIFIC SPORTS EXERCISES
CONDITIONING THROUGH RECREATION

CONDITIONING FOR SPORTS

Physical conditioning is vital to the athlete. It has been repeatedly demonstrated that athletic performance improves after the athlete has conditioned his body in a regular and systematic program of exercise. Moreover, conditioning makes the body less susceptible to injury.

The conditioning program for the athlete consists of two phases: the off-season and the in-season. In the off-season period the concentration in the conditioning program is on achieving and maintaining total body physical fitness. An excellent off-season conditioning program for most athletes would be the Daily Dozen and the Double Dozen coupled with jogging or other endurance-developing exercises. Conditioning in the in-season phase, that is, during the season of participation, is concentrated on bringing the body to top physical condition with special attention directed toward developing those areas of the body on which the sport places the greatest demands. Because all athletic performance requires muscles that are strong and capable of providing sufficient explosive power to perform the necessary tasks, exercises that develop muscular strength and endurance receive major emphasis as do the exercises that develop cardio-respiratory endurance.

Practice sessions and actual game participation do, of course, provide vigorous workouts. Although these are beneficial in conditioning the body, they do not provide complete body exercise and must be supplemented with other conditioning exercises. The daily conditioning program should include running, the Daily Dozen and an abundance of stretching exercises. All can be included in the warm-up session preceding each daily practice.

SPECIFIC SPORTS EXERCISES

The special requirements of each sport are met through specific exercises that are added to the general conditioning program. On the following pages are listed by sports the special requirements and the exercises for each. On the first day of the conditioning program, each exercise should be repeated until fatigue occurs; thereafter, the number of repetitions should be increased gradually until optimum performance is reached.

Badminton, Handball, Squash Racquets and Tennis

Most racquet games require quick movements, changes of direction, pivoting and sudden bursts of speed. Although not a racquet game, handball is included here because of the similarity of the movements involved. Good performance in all these games requires a strong forearm and upper arm. The exercises suggested below will improve playing ability in the listed games and also in such games as paddle tennis, table tennis and deck tennis.

Specific exercises

1. *Rubber ball squeezing:* To develop the strength of the flexors of the fingers and the wrists. Squeeze a rubber ball that fits comfortably in the palm of the hand for five minutes per day. Alternate hands so there will be uniform development in both arms.
2. *Short sprints:* To improve running ability. Run short sprints of 25 yards.
3. *Shuttle run:* To improve agility. Described on page 85.
4. *Cross-overs:* To improve agility. Changing from a spread leg position to a lunge position, bring the left leg over to the right or the right over to the left.
5. *Pivots:* To improve agility. From a spread leg position, cross the right foot over the left. At the same time twist the left foot to turn the body in the opposite direction from the starting position. Repeat to the opposite side.
6. *Isometric exercises* (Nos. 4 to 7): To develop strength of the upper arms and the chest. Described on pages 48 to 51.
7. *Pulley weight exercises:* To develop strength of the upper arms and the chest. Described on pages 72 to 74.

Baseball, Softball and Golf

One portion of the games of baseball and softball involves swinging a bat while another part of the games places sudden demands upon the body and involves quick running movements and jumping. Golf is similar in the sense that swinging a golf club has a relationship to batting and makes like demands on the legs, especially when hilly courses are covered. The hand-eye coordination involved in these games can be improved, mainly by practicing the actual skills of the games, but supplementary exercises are needed to improve arm strength, leg strength and endurance. Running is, of course, the staple exercise for developing cardiorespiratory endurance.

Specific exercises

1. *Pull-ups:* To develop the strength of the flexors of the arms, the wrists and the fingers.
2. *Push-ups:* To develop the extensors of the elbow and strengthen the muscles affecting the shoulder joint (deltoid and pectoralis muscles). Described on pages 17 and 82.
3. *Pulley weight exercise:* To develop the strength of the muscles affecting the shoulder joint (deltoid, latissimus dorsi, trapezius and pectoralis muscles) and the flexors and extensors of the arms and the wrists. The exercise is described on page 73. A bat may be taped to the handle of the pulley weights to provide exercise that simulates the swinging of a bat.
4. *Rubber ball squeezing:* To strengthen the flexors of the fingers. Described on page 99.
5. *Wrist rolls:* To develop the extensors and the flexors of the wrists and the flexors of the fingers. Tape a piece of rope to a bar or stick 18 inches long. On the other end tie a weight of five to ten pounds. Grasp the bar with the palms down. Hold the bar at arm's length and roll the rope up on the bar by turning the bar in the hands. To develop the flexors of the wrists, grasp the bar with the palms up.
6. *Knee bends:* To increase the strength of the thigh muscles (quadriceps). Described on page 60.
7. *Vertical jump:* To increase the explosive power of the extensors of the knees and the ankles. Described on page 79. This test item can be used as an exercise by jumping repeatedly while standing away from the wall and throwing both arms above the head during the jump.

Basketball, Lacrosse and Soccer

These games all involve continuous running, with only short periods of rest during time-out. They also involve quick twisting, pivoting and turning movements that require strong, powerful legs. Basketball and soccer demand vertical jumping ability while basketball and lacrosse require strength of the fingers, the wrists and the arms. The neck muscles of the soccer player must be well developed to meet the demands made on them in heading the ball.

Specific exercises

1. *Short sprints:* To improve running ability. Run short sprints of 25 yards or less.
2. *Vertical jump:* To increase the explosive power of the legs. Described on page 79. This test item can be used as an exercise by jumping repeatedly while standing away from the wall and throwing both arms above the head during the jump.
3. *Knee bends:* To increase the strength of the extensors of the knees. Described on page 60.
4. *Wrist rolls:* To develop the extensors and flexors of the wrists and the flexors of the fingers (for basketball and lacrosse). Described on page 100.
5. *Rubber ball squeezing:* To develop the strength of the flexors of the wrists and the fingers (for basketball and lacrosse). Described on page 99.
6. *Medicine ball throwing:* To develop the chest muscles (pectoralis) and the extensors of the upper arms (for basketball and lacrosse).

    Select a ball suitable for your weight and strength. Eleven-pound balls are usually suitable for those who weigh less than 150 pounds, while 15-pound balls can be used to advantage by those above that weight.

    In a sitting position, face a partner sitting about 15 feet away and hold the ball in both hands above and slightly in back of your head. Throw the ball forward to your partner, extending the wrist and elbow joints. After catching the ball, the partner returns it in a like manner. If you cannot throw it high enough for him to catch it, move closer together.

    The same exercise can be done in a standing position. Take one step forward with each throw. Standing with legs spread wide apart, 15 feet from your partner, begin with the ball held above the head. Swing the ball down between the legs, bring it forward rapidly and then release it quickly in a forward and upward throwing motion. Try to control the ball so that your partner has to reach up to catch it.
7. *Head presses* (sideward, forward, backward): To develop the lateral muscles (sternocleidomastoid) and the extensors and

the flexors of the neck (for soccer). Described on page 55.
8. *Bridging:* To develop the lateral muscles (sternocleidomastoid) and the extensors and the flexors of the neck (for soccer). Take a supine position with the knees bent and the feet on the floor. Bend the head back until it touches the floor. Arch the back and take some of the body's weight on the head. Use the legs to move the body so that the neck is moved back and forth while the head remains stationary on the floor.

Bicycling

Most individuals think of cycling only in terms of the leg action involved in pedaling, which is, of course, the principal action. However, prolonged periods of riding places demands upon the arms, the hands and the fingers that must be met if proper control of the bike is to be maintained.

Specific exercises

1. *Wrist rolls:* To develop the flexors and the extensors of the wrists and the flexors of the fingers. Described on page 100.
2. *Rubber ball squeezing:* To develop the strength of the flexors of the wrists and the fingers. Described on page 99.
3. *Sit-ups:* To develop the strength of the abdominal muscles and the hip flexors. Described on pages 18 and 79.
4. *Knee bends:* To strengthen the extensors of the knee. Described on page 60.
5. *Trunk bends:* To strengthen the muscles of the lower back (erector spinae). Described on page 24.
6. *Stair climbing:* To strengthen the extensors of the knee and the hip. Described on page 96.
7. *Bench stepping:* To strengthen the extensors of the knee and the hip. Described on page 96.

Fencing

The demands of fencing are somewhat different from most sports, yet not unlike those of wrestling, boxing, basketball and soccer, in which feints, changes of pace and sudden aggressive moves are necessary to successful performance. Most of the movement in fencing is either forward or backward, and there is no follow-through in the thrusting movements, but rather a quick withdrawal to be ready for defense. Not all thrusts are necessarily made from a bent-arm position, as might be supposed; many are made with lunging movements which require leg strength and general flexibility.

Specific exercises

1. *Hurdle:* To develop the flexibility of the legs and the hips. Described on page 32.
2. *Pull-ups:* To develop the strength of the flexors of the elbows, wrists and fingers and the extensors of the shoulder joint. Described on page 80.
3. *Push-ups:* To develop the extensors of the elbow and to strengthen the muscles affecting the shoulder joint (deltoid and pectoralis muscles). Described on pages 17 and 82.
4. *Pulley weight exercise:* To develop the strength of the muscles affecting the shoulder joint (deltoid, latissimus dorsi, trapezius and pectoralis muscles) and the flexors and the extensors of the arms and the wrists. Described on page 73.
5. *Wrist rolls:* To develop the strength of the flexors of the fingers. Described on page 100.
6. *Rubber ball squeezing:* To develop the strength of the flexors of the wrists and the fingers. Described on page 99.
7. *Knee bends:* To increase the strength of the extensors of the knee. Described on page 60.
8. *Lunging exercise:* To develop the flexibility of the legs and the hips.
   Do a series of movements like the lunge in fencing without the foil. Stretch as far as possible beyond normal and do the lunges as rapidly as possible.

Football

While other sports demand all-out effort in running, jumping and throwing, no other sport places so varied a demand on strength, speed, skill, agility, balance, flexibility and endurance as the game of football. Strength in football is as essential in the arms, chest, shoulders and back as it is in the legs.

Specific exercises

1. *Endurance training:* To develop cardiorespiratory endurance. Described on pages 90 to 97.
2. *Short sprints:* To improve running ability and to develop cardiorespiratory endurance.

Run short sprints of 25 yards. Walk a few steps and repeat.
3. *Stair climbing:* To develop the endurance and the strength of the ankle, the knee and the hip muscles (quadriceps, hamstrings, gastrocnemius and gluteus maximus muscles). Described on page 96.
4. *Bench stepping:* To develop endurance and strength of the ankles, the knees and the hip muscles (quadriceps, hamstrings, gastrocnemius and gluteus maximus muscles). Described on page 96.
5. *Push-ups:* To develop the extensors of the elbows and to strengthen the muscles affecting the shoulder joint (deltoid and pectoralis muscles). Described on page 17.
6. *Pull-ups:* To develop the strength of the flexors of the elbows, the wrists and the fingers and the extensors of the shoulder joint. Described on page 80.
7. *Pulley weights:* To develop the strength of the muscles affecting the shoulder joint (deltoid, latissimus dorsi, trapezius and pectoralis muscles) and the flexors and the extensors of the elbows and the wrists. Described on page 73.
8. *Medicine ball throwing:* To develop the chest muscles (pectoralis) and the extensors of the upper arm. Described on page 101.
9. *Weight training:* To develop all the major muscle groups of the body.
All of the exercises described on pages 58 to 68 may be used to increase muscle strength.

Gymnastics

Once erroneously thought to be purely an arm and shoulder muscle sport, gymnastics is now considered an activity that demands total physical development. Unlike many sports and games where participation becomes an important conditioning factor, one must be in top physical condition before any of the difficult gymnastic stunts can be performed. Modern gymnastics requires not only strong arm, shoulder and chest muscles, but powerful abdominal and leg muscles as well.

Specific exercises

1. *Pull-ups:* To develop the strength of the flexors of the elbows, the wrists and the fingers and the extensors of the shoulder joint. Described on page 80.

2. *Push-ups:* To develop the extensors of the elbows and to strengthen the muscles of the shoulder joint (deltoid and pectoralis muscles). Described on pages 17 and 82.
3. *Dips:* To develop the extensors of the elbows and the flexors of the shoulder joint.

    Parallel bars are necessary for this exercise. Take a front support position, grasp the bars and jump up between the bars. Take the weight of the body on the arms, keeping them straight. Then lower the body until the upper arms are parallel to the floor. Return to original position and repeat.
4. *Bent arm hang and one-half lever at hips:* To develop the flexors of the elbows and the hips and the abdominal flexors and shoulder extensors.

    Take a position on a bar with the elbows bent at a 90 degree angle. Raise both legs at the hips until they are parallel to the floor and hold the position.

Ice Hockey

Speed, change in direction, change of pace, strong arms and shoulders and endurance are all necessary to play hockey well. The same may be said of other sports, but most of these are contested on firm footing. Balance, which is also necessary in other sports, is further complicated in skating by the slippery ice and the narrow runners and the stilt effect of the skates.

General conditioning for hockey need not be different from that for football except for extra stress on the legs, the ankles and the feet. Skating can, of course, be substituted for running. Some coaches do not approve of their players running, but there is no proof that running has any adverse effect upon skating prowess.

Groin injuries are a skater's nemesis. Exercises involving leg adduction, abduction, flexion and extension will help to prevent such injuries.

Specific exercises

1. *Chop chop* (cross arms and legs): To develop hip flexors, abductors and adductors. Described on page 23.
2. *Isometric exercise for hips:* To develop the muscles that abduct the hips. Described on page 52.
3. *Leg abductor and adductor exercise:* To develop the abductors and adductors of the hips.

    Stand with each foot on a separate towel or similar material (the floor beneath must be slippery). Hold on to a bar, chair

or table. Begin with the legs spread and draw the feet together. Take some of the weight on the hands while doing this. Next, push the feet apart, and then repeat the exercise. Begin with the feet only slightly apart at first, and when the movement becomes easier, increase the distance.
4. *Hip extensor and flexor exercise:* To develop the extensor and the flexor muscles of the hips.

    The exercise performed above may also be used in a forward and back sliding action. Bending the knee of the forward leg and extending the leg that is back will also aid in stretching the ligaments.
5. *Ankle flexion and extension exercise:* To develop the flexors and the extensors of the ankles.

    Stand with toes and balls of feet on a board and with a weighted bar across the back and shoulders, and begin with the heels on the floor. Rise up slowly on the toes until the heels are well above the level of the board. Lower them slowly and repeat. Add or take off weight, depending upon your own individual capacity to perform the exercise.

Skiing

Skiing, whether it is downhill, cross-country or jumping, involves strong action by the legs with some assist from the arms in maintaining balance and using the poles. Conditioning exercises for skiing must emphasize the development of strength in the hips, the legs and the ankles.

Specific exercises

1. *Stair climbing:* To strengthen the extensors of the knees and the hips. Described on page 96.
2. *Bench stepping:* To strenthen the extensors of the knees and the hips. Described on page 96.
3. *Knee bends:* To strengthen the extensors of the knees and the ankles. Described on page 60.
4. *Ankle flexion and extension exercise:* To develop the strength of the lower leg muscles (gastrocnemius and tibialis anterior). Described on pages 69 and 70.
5. *Chop chop* (cross arms and legs): To develop the thigh flexors, abductors and adductors. Described on page 23.
6. *Isometric exercise for the hips:* To develop the muscles that abduct the legs. Described on page 52.
7. *Leg adductor and abductor exercise:* To develop the adductors and abductors of the legs. Described on pages 52 to 54.

Swimming

Once considered by many professional people to be the perfect form of exercise, training for swimming today would seem to refute this idea. Many swimming coaches have been turning to work with weights in order to give their men more strength. Bob Kiphuth, whose swimming teams' won-lost dual meet records stand above those of any other swim team, pioneered the use of preseason body building programs to prepare his men for the long swim season. Continued repetition of the same exercise was his prescription. His Yale team record of 528 wins as against only 12 losses, two of which were against nonintercollegiate teams, speaks for itself.

Specific exercises

1. *Double Dozen:* To develop the strength of the total body. Described on pages 15 to 42.
2. *Pulley weight exercise:* To develop the strength of the muscles affecting the shoulder joint (deltoid, latissimus dorsi, trapezius and pectoralis muscles) and the flexors and the extensors of the arms and the wrists. Described on page 73.
3. *Medicine ball throwing:* To develop the chest muscles (pectoralis) and the extensors of the upper arms. Described on page 101.
4. *Ankle stretcher* (flexion): To increase the flexibility of the ankle. Described on page 69.
5. *Ankle stretcher* (extension): To increase flexibility of the ankle. Described on page 70.
6. *Shoulder stretcher:* To increase the flexibility of the shoulders. Described on page 71.
7. *Arm and leg stretch:* To increase flexibility of the shoulders and the legs. Described on page 72.

Track and Field

The number of different events in a track program precludes any possibility of covering each one in detail here. Basically, the exercises for running and jumping should stress strengthening the leg muscles and developing cardiorespiratory endurance. The exercises for the throwing events should also stress these and should include in addition the development of strength in the arms, the hands and the shoulders.

Specific exercises

1. *Endurance training:* To develop cardiorespiratory endurance. Described on pages 90 to 97.

2. *Vertical jump:* To strengthen the leg muscles. Described on page 79.
3. *Knee bends:* To increase the strength of the extensors of the knees and the ankles. Described on page 60.
4. *Stair climbing:* To strengthen the extensors of the knees and the hips. Described on page 96.
5. *Hurdle:* To develop the flexibility of the legs and the hips. Described on page 32.
6. *Ankle flexion and extension exercise:* To develop the strength of the lower leg muscles (gastrocnemius and tibialis anterior). Described on pages 69 and 70.
7. *Pulley weight exercises:* To develop the strength of the muscles affecting the shoulder joint (deltoid, latissimus dorsi, trapezius, pectoralis muscles) and the flexors and the extensors of the arms and the wrists. Described on page 73.
8. *Pull-ups:* To develop the strength of the flexors of the elbows, the wrists and the fingers and the extensors of the shoulder joint. Described on page 80.
9. *Push-ups:* To develop the strength of the muscles affecting the shoulder joint (deltoid and pectoralis muscles) and the extensors of the elbows. Described on pages 17 and 82.
10. *Dips:* To develop the extensors of the elbow and the muscles affecting the shoulder joint (latissimus and pectoralis muscles). Described on page 81.

Volleyball

Agility and explosiveness are the physical attributes most needed by volleyball players. In addition, much stretching and twisting are involved. Finger and wrist strength are important to successful ball handling.

Specific exercises

1. *Vertical jump:* To increase the explosive power of the extensors of the knees and the ankles. Described on page 79.
2. *Knee bends:* To increase the strength of the extensors of the knees. Described on page 60.
3. *Ankle flexion and extension exercise:* To develop the strength of the lower leg muscles (gastrocnemius and tibialis anterior). Described on pages 69 and 70.
4. *Wrist rolls:* To develop the extensors and the flexors of the wrists and the flexors of the fingers. Described on page 100.
5. *Rubber ball squeezing:* To develop the strength of the flexors of the wrists and the fingers. Described on page 99.

6. *Twister:* To increase the elasticity of the hamstring muscles of the leg as well as the flexibility of the back. Described on page 16.

Wrestling

Wrestling requires a constant effort to improve upon one's overall physical attributes. If both wrestlers are equally skillful during competition, strength can decide the winner. To best your opponent in strength means that you must have more endurance than he, and if strength and endurance are equal, quickness and agility can be the deciding factors in a match.

Specific exercises

1. *Bridging:* To develop the lateral muscles (sternocleidomastoid) and the extensors and the flexors of the neck. Described on page 102.
2. *Weight training exercises:* To develop the strength of the total body. Described on pages 58 to 68.
3. *Rubber ball squeeze:* To develop the strength of the wrists and the fingers. Described on page 99.
4. *Sit-ups:* To develop the strength of the abdominal muscles and the hip flexors. Described on page 18.
5. *Flexibility exercises:* To develop the flexibility of the total body. Described on pages 68 to 72.

CONDITIONING THROUGH RECREATION

Participation in sports for recreation can serve as an important part of a conditioning program if the participation is strenuous and frequent. Recreational sports, however, are usually engaged in only during weekend leisure time. Weekend playing, even when extremely vigorous, cannot be considered sufficient to achieve and maintain good physical condition. As has been repeatedly pointed out, regular workouts throughout the week are necessary to accomplish this.

Those enthusiasts for certain sports who play daily or nearly every day can expect improved physical fitness. The amount of improvement will be determined by the strenuousness of the game and the completeness of the exercise that it provides. Very vigorous sports such as touch football will effect a greater amount of improvement

Table 4. Some Recommended Sports Activities

The Young
Vigorous Participation

Aquatic sports	Hiking
Canoeing	Hockey—field
Fishing—game	—ice
Scuba diving	Horseback riding
Skin diving	Lacrosse
Swimming—speed	Rowing
—distance	Skating—ice
—recreational	—roller
Badminton	Skiing
Baseball	Soccer
Bicycling	Squash racquets
Dancing	Tennis
Football—tackle	Track and field
Gymnastics	Volleyball (two-man)
Handball	Wrestling

The Middle Years
Moderate Approach

Aquatic sports	Football—touch
Boating	Golf
Canoeing	Gymnastics
Fishing—casting	Handball
—trolling	Hiking
—game	Rowing
Scuba diving	Skating—ice
Skin diving	—roller
Swimming—recreational	Squash racquets
Badminton	Tennis
Bicycling	Volleyball
Dancing	

Senior Citizens
More Moderate Participation

Aquatic sports	Bowling
Boating	Curling
Canoeing	Dancing
Fishing—casting	Golf—limited no. of holes
—still	Hiking—moderation
—trolling	Ping-pong—volley game
Sailing	Shuffle board
Swimming—recreational	Skating—leisurely
Archery	Walking

than milder games such as golf and bowling. No game provides total body exercise, but some do so more completely than others; tennis, for example, provides more complete exercise than shuffleboard.

It is not intended that this discussion of the limitations of recreational sports and games should discourage participation in them. They offer opportunities for sociability and relaxation that everyone should have and their use as leisure activity is extremely worthwhile. Rather, the intent is to point up the need to engage in a conditioning program in addition to recreational play.

As people grow older, the kinds of recreational sports and games in which they engage must change because the body becomes less able to adapt to activity. Possibilities for recreational sports for different age groups are suggested in Table 4. It should be pointed out that those who have maintained a high level of physical fitness throughout the years will remain more adaptable than those who have not.

GLOSSARY

A.A.H.P.E.R.—American Association for Health, Physical Education and Recreation.
Abduction—Movement away from the midline of the body.
Adduction—Movement toward the midline of the body.
Aerobic—Living or active only in the presence of oxygen.
A.M.A.—American Medical Association.
Antagonistic—In anatomical nomenclature, refers to muscles of opposite action.
Atherosclerosis—A form of arteriosclerosis in which the arteries are lined with small drops of fat.
Calorie—The amount of heat required to raise the temperature of 1 kilogram of water 1° centigrade. Used to express the energy-producing value of foods.
Cardiorespiratory—Refers to the heart and the lungs and the exchange of oxygen from the lungs into the circulatory system.
Cholesterol—A fatty substance in the circulatory system, carried through the blood.
Circuit training—The arrangement of an exercise program done in a specific order. Two alternatives given include a set number of repetitions done as rapidly as possible, or a set time in which as many repetitions as possible can be done.
Depression—Movement of the arms downward from any point between an overhead position and the hips.
Elevation—Movement of the arms to an overhead position.
Extension—The straightening of a joint.
Flexibility—The ability to achieve maximum movement in all joints of the body.
Flexion—The act of bending. This term can be associated with all joints of the body.
Isometric—Exercise involving movement against, or resistance from, an immovable object, pitting one muscle group against another.
Isotonic—Exercise involving free movement.
Position—The situation or state in which a person is set or placed in order to begin an exercise.
Primary—The term used to describe muscles that cause a specific movement by their action or contraction.
Prone—Body in horizontal position with face down.
Rests—Rests are positions held in an exercise. Leaning rest refers to a position in which the body is held rigid, with only the hands and feet touching the floor. In a front leaning rest position, the chest is toward the floor,

with only the hands and toes touching. A back leaning rest is done with the back toward the floor and only the hands and heels touching. A side leaning rest is held with the side of the body toward the floor and only one hand and the side of the foot on the floor.

Rotation — Moving on an axis.

Secondary — The term used to describe certain muscles not directly causing a movement, but which lend support to that movement.

Shoulder girdle — The shoulder girdle is made up of two bones, the scapular bones in back and the clavicular bones in front below the neck. The clavicular bones are joined by the sternum in front, while both bones come together and with the arm bone form the shoulder joint.

Supine — Body in horizontal position with face up.

Visceral — Pertaining to the internal organs, especially those in the abdominal cavity.

BIBLIOGRAPHY

Bowen and McKenzie: *Applied Anatomy and Kinesiology.* 5th ed. Revised by Boughner and Rynearson. Philadelphia, Lea & Febiger, 1944. This is a well-written and well-illustrated text, with good, clear explanations and many excellent illustrations.

Doherty, J. Kenneth: *Modern Track and Field.* 2nd ed. Englewood Cliffs, N.J., Prentice-Hall, Inc., 1963. One of the most complete and authoritative texts written on a particular sport. Mr. Doherty blends the knowledge gained from his experience as an athlete and coach with the experiences of other fine coaches and athletes into an extremely well-organized and detailed text.

Dyson, Geoffrey: *The Mechanics of Athletics.* 2nd ed. London, The University of London Press, 1963. A fresh approach to the mechanics involved in sport, with excellent descriptions and illustrations.

Karpovich, Peter V.: *Physiology of Muscular Activity.* 6th ed. Philadelphia, W. B. Saunders Company, 1965. A basic text for the understanding of the nature of muscles and their functions. It includes material as varied as the role of oxygen in physical exertion, the "Relation Between Physical Fitness and Intelligence" and "The Functions of Organs for Muscular Work." Both sides of debatable topics are presented, which makes the book unique in this field.

Kranz, Leon: *Kinesiology Manual.* 3rd ed. St. Louis, The C. V. Mosby Co., 1956. Excellent descriptions of the many variations in human movement, and exercises with drawings. A fine analysis of the action of individual muscles as well as the action caused by muscle groups.

Massey, Benjamin H., et al.: *The Kinesiology of Weight Training.* Dubuque, Iowa, Wm. C. Brown Co., 1959. A well-illustrated, comprehensive analysis and description of weight training and weight lifting. The various movements, the muscles involved, and the objectives are set forth in detail for almost every type of exercise involving use of weights.

The Research Quarterly, 1201 16th St., N.W., Washington, D.C. A publication of the American Association for Health, Physical Education and Recreation. Many excellent scientific studies on physical education activities, sports and athletics appear in this publication.